THE ULTIMATE VEGAN DIET FOR WOMEN

2021 EDITION

contents

demonstration

What is this herbal diet?

What is the difference?

Are Vegetarian Diets the Best Solution?

What about vitamin B12?

What happens to omega-3 fatty acids?

FOOD-PRINTER

PLANTS AND HEALTH

PLANTS AND COMMON INFLAMMATION

SNEAKY TIP TO LOSE WEIGHT UNCERTAINTY

Plants and other benefits

Would meals be as good as used to?

THE DIFFERENCE BETWEEN THE FOOD AND THE PLANT PLAN

FOODS

FOOD DESIGN BUILDING GUIDE

Live plans

ESTABLISHING BUILDING SERVICES The 50 most important food principles

cash receipts

demonstration

Like most people who change plants, I wondered if food would be sufficient. Moreover, I am worried to find inspirational and restrictive vegetarian food, mostly in the belief that the plant Œ Vegetarian show ± food boring and tasteless are wit petal. Worked namely em wi ê c little ê teach ® ê how to make healthy foods on the planet. I followed the chef's training in an intuitive vegetable-based kitchen, which included learning how to cook according to the chef's intuition, without recipes. Because I wanted to make sure I had everything my body needed, I went back to school to learn the nutrition I needed, focusing on the natural approach to a healthy lifestyle.

I've never had such fun cooking and eating before. I never feel restricted or private; and conversely, I feel free, discovering endless possibilities through new flavors and combinations of flavors and constantly adding new and interesting foods and foods to my list of recipes. After switching to a lifestyle based on the plants I have more energy; I lost weight without trying; and I have no chronic problems with gas or digestion. I've had it before. I didn't realize how bad I felt until I felt better.

This is how my path to plants evolved, but I know that every path is different because our eating experiences are different. The way we eat is very personal. Food not only nourishes our bodies, it also has the power to make life more enjoyable. Food is closely related to culture and social life, and our taste buds force us to seek happiness and satisfaction in food. Maintaining a herbal lifestyle can be difficult in flesh and comfort in a full society. Most people are afraid of the idea of stopping eating and learning to make new and bizarre foods with those who know little or nothing and who sometimes cannot even utter. And if you eat plants, it's not natural, it's hard to get caught up in countless vegan cookbooks and blogs and rely on existing plants.

Here the book is different. The food plan and recipes in this book are designed to teach you how to cook the best vegetable dishes so that the meal itself is an incentive. As for plants, regardless of the transition reason, just add more vegetables in the diet, lose ten pounds of stubborn, show thin from this special evening event, make long-term health changes l HCl k s instructions rin l ö co HCl up being relief   and symptoms of chronic diseases or the like min s , hiilijalanj s ljen v s hent s a v s hent s m s ll s meat and dairy products; In fact, if sy o m s si taste of food does her ä tt HCl to you, you can not eat this way for up to three weeks.

I decided to equip myself with culinary training, but it is not far from the success of this diet. Using the knowledge and techniques that have helped me and many of my clients, I have carefully developed these recipes to explore a variety of dishes for quick and easy meals using, which is hy o ty s ty o n j s after that busy or s y o n s . I am inspired by my o s round the ä the globe are located in the appliance o t, so I l ö co HCl new favorite food, cooking or recipe, expanding vocabulary and culinary experiences. In addition, the three-week Meal Program includes daily menus and shopping lists that will show you exactly how to make this diet work for you and help you stay on track. You'll find a clear guide and a solid plan of action for a fully nutritious vegan diet that constantly focuses on delicious and healthy foods. You can also prepare meals that meat lovers will love.

Finally, the great thing about eating and enjoying plants is that after three weeks you start to see and feel their healing power. Your hip is radiant, your digestion improves, you have more energy, you think better and you sleep better. If you have been following this diet for a long time, you should find that your immune system is more robust, your mood is more balanced, your life is slimmer and your mind is calming as you make decisions.

What is this herbal diet?

All vegetarian foods and diets are sometimes referred to as the WFPB diet; Although many nutritionists and doctors have differences in the list of vegetarian diets, there is one thing that everyone agrees: a vegetable or WFPB diet is more than just a diet. First of all, it is a way of life.

It is a way of life that means different things to different people because people also define what is a vegetarian diet for them, while some people leave room for animal products such as eggs and milk; others choose not to leave any type of animal food.

However, most herbal diets have certain features that make them generally accepted by nutritionists, doctors, and individuals. These functions are

- The food you focus on is mainly plants such as vegetables, fruits, legumes, seeds, whole grains and nuts.
- Are animal products completely restricted or prohibited (depending on the person)
- This diet helps to focus on the quality of the food we consume, and many Vegetarian Diet Followers are 100% organic and derived from local sources.
- All vegetable food preparations are complete without any transformation (or very v s h s of the change in MIK s li possible)

These root causes mean that this diet is sometimes mistaken for a vegan or vegetarian diet; Even though they have similarities, they still have their own characteristics.

What is the difference?

Vegan Diets: People who follow a vegan diet keep away from all animal products such as crustaceans, honey, meat, eggs, milk, and poultry.

Vegetarians: There are two types of vegetarians; There are those who eat dairy products, shellfish. There are also vegetarians who remove poultry and meat from their diet.

Herbal diet: Herbal diet is quite flexible. Many fans consume plant-based foods, but el s intuotteet EIV s t not possibly deadly taboo (though some consider). Some sy o v s t t s completely planned diet, others sy o v s s milk, eggs, poultry, meat and s compa s dad s .

Plant or plant diets (as some call it) are diets that focus on healthy herbal foods.

Are Vegetarian Diets the Best Solution?

Some people had reason to ask me if plant diets are a really good option because there are also health benefits that can be obtained from other sources.

That is true, but you have nothing to lose if you follow a purely vegetarian diet.

Vegetarian foods provide you with essential nutrients such as vitamins, fats, proteins, minerals and carbohydrates to ensure a healthy diet and body, as well as plenty of nutrients and fiber. For those who bypass all forms of animal products in their diet, they need to take in certain nutrients, such as B12, so that their bodies receive all the nutrients they need.

Some people said they like this diet, but my options are limited.

There is no bigger lie than that. Did you know that you can make cocktails, purees, pizzas and other delicious and delicious foods that make your palate more desirable? Plus, they are all healthy and nutritious plant products! You can't do it better.

Even if you continue with this diet, you can be sure that your food contains all the nutrients you need, even if it is a herbal diet. Herbal products ensure that your body lacks the minerals needed for body development and growth.

What about vitamin B12?

Vitamin B12 is an essential nutrient that the body needs to make blood cells and nerves active and healthy. This vitamin allows the body to protect itself from a severe anemia called megaloblastic anemia and to renew its body. not wear out easily and not get tired People with low levels of vitamin B12 can get weaker due to fatigue.

This particular vitamin is one of the few vitamins to be obtained from animal products; You will find dairy products like milk or margarine. If you are using a plant-based diet that does not contain animal products, you can easily get tired or faint.

A good way to get this vitamin is by taking vitamin B in the form of nutritional supplements.

Don't worry, even people who do not use herbs, such as the elderly, pregnant women's diets and other people who have vitamin B deficiency take these supplements with age because the body has problems absorbing this vitamin because your doctor may prescribe this drug .

What happens to omega-3 fatty acids?

Omega-3 fatty acids are very important for the body. It is known to help the body fight inflammation, increase body resistance and prevent autoimmune diseases, prevent cancer, help mental health, relieve anxiety and depression, and help the brain develop fetuses, prevent Alzheimer's disease, reduce the risk of childhood ADHD and asthma.

Omega-3 fatty acids are usually found in blue fish (in large amounts), but that does not mean they are not found in other seeds and nuts. If you are on a plant-based diet, you can get it from other sources like hemp seeds, nuts, soybeans, chia seeds, ground flax seeds, flax seeds and their oils. Omega-3 fatty acids are also found in algae oil and fennel oil

FOOD-PRINTER

Before we move on to balanced meal plans and delicious recipes, we study and understand the principles and learning of herbal diets. You can get started, but in the long run, you should find out why and what we do. It saves you time by starting to understand how to prepare a balanced and delicious meal instead of always following your plans and recipes. Chapter one looks at the relationship between herbal diet and health; then we move on to a balanced distribution of plant nutrition; Then I will give you many tips and tips for setting herbal food.

PLANTS AND HEALTH

Unfortunately, chronic conditions such as cancer and heart disease are very common in the United States. There is good evidence that changing eating habits can help prevent chronic diseases, and a diet rich in meat and dairy products is associated with major health problems such as heart disease and diabetes. Many meats and dairy compounds (such as casein, nitrite, saturated fat, cholesterol, heme iron and arachidonic acid) are considered to be possible culprits for this combination.

All of this has sparked a growing interest in plant diets for health reasons, as vegetarian foods are a rich source of nutrients and compounds that help protect us from chronic diseases. Before discussing what to eat to support this new lifestyle, you should look more closely at the role of plants in controlling weight loss and promoting a healthier life.

Plants as a medicine

One of the most important choices that you can do for your health is to eat more fresh fruits and vegetables, whole jyvi s , beans, p ä nut o it s , melon seeds ä , herbs ä and spices. By integrating more th s s s s IT s products el s m HCl Si has a strong effect.

Herbal diets are high in dietary fiber, magnesium, folic acid, vitamins C and E, iron and phytochemicals. They also have a lower calorific value and they are   less saturated fat and cholesterol than other diets. Vegetarians are generally less at risk for cardiovascular disease, obesity, type 2 diabetes and certain cancers.

heart disease

Heart disease is the leading cause of death for Americans. Dietary recommendations for people at risk of cardiovascular disease include decreased saturated fat, cholesterol, purified carbohydrates and sugar, and increased fiber, antioxidants, omega-3 and polyunsaturated fats. The best way to do this is to eat a vegetarian diet (eating vegetables, whole grains, nuts, seeds, pulses and fruits).

In studies, vegans have lower cardiovascular disease than carnivores and even vegetarians: low blood pressure, low LDL cholesterol (low type), low triglyceride levels, low total serum cholesterol and apolipoprotein B (transported cholesterol) and lipoproteins and people with vascular disease, reduce systolic and diastolic blood pressure, and reduce the incidence of hypertension.

Vegetarians are generally less likely to have hypertension, probably because of the high consumption of potassium in vegetables, fruits, grains and legumes. Blood pressure is related to the percentage of sodium in relation to body potassium. Although the general recommendation for people with high blood pressure is to reduce salt intake, it has not been shown to significantly affect blood pressure control. Another key to this equation is to add the potassium side of the compound. The average consumption of a typical American is 2: 1, which means that Potasie has twice ê more sodium than desired this is for the data. The ideal ratio is 1: 5, so æ c reduction of salt (sodium chloride), so not enough ± . In order to increase the potassium balance, it is necessary to eat more herbal foods.

A plant-based diet significantly increases the yield of protective nutrients (such as antioxidants) and phytochemicals (compounds of plants that are useful to us) by minimizing the intake of high-risk compounds associated with various chronic diseases. This does not mean that vegans are immune to this disease: heredity and other environmental and lifestyle factors are also involved. But a herbal diet offers the best ways to avoid risk and help build a strong immune system to cope with all the challenges you can't control.

tumor

Cancer is the second leading cause of death in the United States. Whole plant foods as close to natural state as possible contain high levels of potent antioxidants to combat cancer and nutrients that strengthen the immune system, and naturally have low levels of saturated fat and fiber, much more legumes (seeds), peas and beans), more fruits and vegetables, more fiber and more vitamin C than all foods. These foods and their nutrients have proven to be particularly protective against cancer. The plant-based diet also reduces foods with an increased risk of cancer, including dairy products, eggs, red meat and processed meat.

Stroke risk factors are the same as the heart s n disease: high cholesterol, hypertension and obesity. Because the herbal diet improves all three, it is a good way to balance the risk.

Alzheimer's disease and dementia

Although the onset of Alzheimer's disease and dementia is mainly due to heredity, a nutrient-rich vegetable diet provides the best chance for our body to stay healthy as long as possible. One of the factors that can accelerate the occurrence of dementia is oxidative stress, an imbalance between the amount of free radicals in the body and the ability to neutralize damage by neutralizing damage (free radicals damage membranes. Cells and other structures, including DNA). Plants are the richest source of antioxidants in the diet and can help reduce these damage.

Recommendations for delaying the onset and development of Alzheimer's disease often include eating fish and shellfish when it comes to omega-3 fatty acids. However, the study also shows that toxins, heavy metals, and nerve cells are C-nerve cells that promote neurodegeneration. Since fish and seafood, will inevitably have a wealth of mercury and other toxins polluting the oceans, such as plastic, such as plastic, it makes more sense to look for the primary omega-3 acids sources, such as linseed and chiaa.

One of the first questions is when people say that their parents start to show signs of dementia if they get enough vitamin B and folic acid. Lack of these ingredients causes symptoms that mimic dementia. Folic acid can easily be obtained from vegetarian foods, but the density of nutrients needed to maintain a healthy body and mind is not always a priority in our diet. As the metabolism of the elderly slows down, they need more and less. As we age, our bodies can get less vitamin B their diet, make recommendations to the government that over 50 people take supplements B , or they do not consume animal products.

diabetes

The most important dietary recommendations for diabetes are to reduce glycemic load (the overall dietary potential raises blood glucose levels) and saturated fat intake, to increase fiber intake and to use cinnamon. It has been studied for possible benefits in controlling blood glucose levels . This can be easily achieved with a plant-based diet. Many people with pre- and type-2 diabetes have found that their blood sugar levels are much easier to control as they want the floating food they want - Linn's diet.

PLANTS AND COMMON INFLAMMATION

Studies of the relationship between arthritis and diet have shown that people on a plant-based diet significantly reduce morning stiffness, joint pain, swelling and inflammatory compounds in the blood. This is probably due to the fact that the plant diet increases the consumption of anti-inflammatory foods and reduces the consumption of inflammatory compounds from food of animal origin. In infected pigs, there may also be a link with bacteria called Yersinia, which can cause chronic inflammation. Even worse, vegans tend to have lower body weight than meat eaters, which puts less pressure on the joints.

FOODS INFLAMMED

Meat, fish and eggs are a rich source of arachidonic acid, a precursor to inflammatory compounds (prostaglandins and leukotrienes). A low arachidonic acid diet has been shown to relieve the symptoms of arthritis. Advanced glycation end products (AGEs) are inflammatory toxins that occur when food is heated, cooked, baked, or pasteurized. They are mainly formed in animal feeds because the reaction is caused by saturated proteins and fats. They also occur in our bodies when we eat too much sugar and refined flour. Dairy products are one of the most common causes of joint pain because they contain protein that can irritate the tissue around the joints.

Foods to reduce inflammation.

Naturally, all vegetarian foods are rich in anti-inflammatory compounds such as fiber, water, and antioxidants, and of course, all of the inflammatory compounds listed on the left are missing. The main NSAIDs are yellow, red, orange and green leafy vegetables rich in carotenoids such as spinach, cabbage and cabbage, nuts rich in polyunsaturated fats such as almonds and walnuts, or flaxseed. - 3, fruits such as strawberries, berries, cherries and pineapple containing anthocyanins, rich in bromelain, turmeric (due to curcumin) and ginger (due to ginger compounds).

Slimming plants

Despite our dedication to counting calories, going step by step, going to the gym and following diets that eliminate everything we love, or adding a "miracle" nutrition, obesity and disease drift are increasingly affecting our society. Poor nutrition is not an effective long-term strategy, and calorie restriction slows down metabolism, which makes weight loss more difficult.

Thinking about food in terms of nutrient density and calories is a simpler and more effective way to combat weight loss. You can lose weight by adding more nutrient-dense foods and reducing junk food. The magic of this approach is that it changes the focus on creating positive health for you by eating tastier and more satisfying things.

Nutritional foods are high in vitamins, minerals and antioxidants. Vegetables, fruits, whole grains, beans, herbs and spices are foods rich in nutrients. High calorie foods have a high calorie content. Some examples are oils, sugars, dairy products, eggs, blue fish, meat and fried foods.

There are many nutrient- and calorie-rich foods like nuts, seeds and avocados. You want to eat these products because they contain minerals and other important nutrients and small amounts can help you feel full. You should eat them only in smaller portions than other foods rich in nutrients.

Some products do not contain nutrients, even if they do increase calories a day. These are called empty calories. Let your body want nutrients even if you are adding calories to your day. Examples are white rice, white bread, refined oils and refined sugar.

Owning plants and focusing on all foods instead of complex or sophisticated versions increases nutrient density by reducing calorie density. It also increases the consumption of water and fiber, increasing metabolism and improving digestion.

All elements of the diet work together for deep body comfort and nutrition, which naturally develops through dieting. Over time, you will find that these powerful cravings for cheap food will simply disappear because you feel energy and health are rising. Add and develop, don't deny or delete, so that you feel rich, happy and happy.

SNEAKY TIP TO LOSE WEIGHT UNCERTAINTY

Use Bowls and Small Plates With a large plate or bowl, most people take larger portions to visually fill the space. Use the same size plates and bowls at all meals to learn how to fill them with portions that you over-eat during the day.

Use only two or three flavors Our taste buds and brains handle the senses of different tastes during a meal and want to experience a certain amount before we feel satisfied. If we have too many different dishes and flavors at the same time, sy o mme tend s more th s n as needed, so that everyone can taste the well. Example T s st s k s handbook is. So if we prepare a meal consisting of only two or three different meals, we are satisfied before the filling is complete.

Eat chopsticks. It slows down (most of us) and produces small bites, which gives us a better chance of feeling perfect in the body before eating too much.

Swallow between each bite. It's harder than it sounds! Try to check if you are aware of chewing. It also slows down the signs of satiety slightly.

Brushing your teeth between meals This is a great idea for oral hygiene and also reduces the risk of accidental eating between meals. Fuel and nutrient snacks are obviously a good idea, but it's best to minimize unnecessary bites.

Changing the Caloric Density of **Food** When you cook brown rice with another glass of water, the calorie density will decrease. It will be the same, just a little . You can also do this in the morning to get more hydration to start the day; In addition, it is easier to blend.

Diluting Juice or Soda One of the most effective ways to lose a few pounds with a change is to replace juice or soda with water. You can drink lots of sugar, up to 100% natural fruit juice, without knowing how many calories you've added to your day. Can't you go cold turkey? Start by diluting the drinks with water or non-alcoholic drinks. Halving them will reduce sugar consumption . Dilute gradually until you need a little flavor in sparkling water or gas.

Plants and other benefits

There are many other potential health benefits of eating multiple plants. Here are some that people found when switching to a herbal diet.

Pick up and exchange **energy** nutrient-rich vegetarian foods that provide energy levels, lots of sugars and refined grains, which will inevitably raise your blood sugar, and many people know.

Facial cleansing: Dairy products are one of the most common and clearly related factors of acne. Sugar is also a common trigger, so when you lower your refined sugars and switch to whole grain sweets, your skin is likely to be cleansed.

Increased Immunity The nutrients your immune system needs are rich in plants. Focus on dark green, red and orange fruits and vegetables and zinc seeds.

Better Digestion With high fiber growth, many people find that their **digestion** improves. Many of my turtle clients thought the pants were better because they had a smaller stomach.

Belly to soothe too much meat, dairy products, products and fatty foods, poor chewing and stress can make use of the s -section of the magical and the culprits s n s r s stykseen and ruoansulatush s iri ö in.

Faster recovery after training Athletes, runners, and bodybuilders who use a percentage of a plant-based diet that quickly renews after training,

The result: If you can be healthy and to feed the herbal diet, reduce the risk of devastating neurodegenerative diseases, help the planet, el s ame s and animal husbandry k s rsimyksi days as well as days sy ö interesting and nutritious dishes. others with incredible taste: who is still the reason not to change?

Would meals be as good as used to?

I assure you that the vegetable diet is not limited to the vegetarian diet (although leafy vegetables are quite important). The truth is that many times the same vegetables are not ± able to provide ® sufficient ± smokers in quantities to improve performance.

It's a combination

• Fruits like apples, bananas, strawberries, oranges, berries, etc. This is also your favorite fruit .

• Vegetables such as carrots, lettuce, cabbage, broccoli, cabbage, you can also add the vegetables you want to this list.

• Whole grains such as barley, millet, oats, wheat, quinoa etc.

• Pulses such as lentils, chick peas, black beans, etc.

• Tubers, such as potatoes, corn, peas etc. to mention other can become excellent and delicious specialties.

You will be surprise a variety of delicious dishes, delicious j s dessert and even wholesome s v s instance, fire, that you can still sy o d s t s m s s el s m s in accordance with the ntavan. So I can say that s meals EIV s t would be boring HCl or boring HCl , even if you had to give up some suosikkiruoista and snacks.

Most of the ajastaasi amylaceouos focuses on foods that are dependent on it and which it has been for generations.

Consider creating products like black beans, corn, peas, potatoes, brown rice, quinoa, beans and even chick peas. They would be prepared differently, but most of these foods are what you know and you can try them with your meals. Sweet potato lasagna, mashed potatoes and salsa, black beans and rice burrito that you can eat as much as you want with whole fruits

Talking about what you want to eat is also a benefit of vegetarian food, you don't have to worry about counting calories or controlling your doses. Vegetarian diets have a high volume that contains more fiber and water, and this space takes up more space, then fills up the stomach and removes hunger, even if you've consumed less calories than a regular burger.

Some people who follow this diet sometimes worry about eating some type of green vegetables, calcium, beans for protein, nuts for fat; You have to give up that mentality, because the key to this lifestyle is the choice of food for the whole plant you want.

Within a short period of time, many practical foods, such as hamburgers, potatoes, or fast food, will appear.

Can you maintain this lifestyle?

Yes, yes and yes ä !!! It is always and still is, my answer t s h s of the question.

Experts agree that limiting processed and refined foods, such as eating your own foods, ordering your favorite foods, and replacing them with herbs, is beneficial to the body.

When you start a herbal diet, you will see first-hand results like lower blood pressure and lower cholesterol, lower medications, adaptability to old clothes, and even find that it is better to sleep at night and get up fresh in the morning. Become!

However, you are wondering how to motivate yourself to continue? If the results you see are not enough for you and you are starting to overcome obstacles, know that you have several ways to navigate and move towards a healthy lifestyle.

You can achieve this lifestyle in a number of ways, some of which are;

1.   First of all, be your motivation

If you want, you can pursue this lifestyle as an assistant and encourage yourself by setting goals that you intend to achieve. Set up the records yourself and work on decrypting them. For example, suppose you wanted to run a dog from a distance and not run out of breath or a marathon, wear old clothes or clothing of a certain size. Save your progress on an award-winning magazine and movie. I can also write notes that I can read later to encourage him and tell him how he's doing.

2.   Let others inspire you

If success is not enough, let someone inspire you. Videos about people who are dieting and telling about their success can also help you stay focused and remember that you have decided to do it.

See how it works for others. It can help you stay on track and stay motivated.

3.   Never stop learning

Read books (like this one) on healthy eating, natural cookbooks, expert guides or nutrition books, which can also be inspirational. Learning something new about this lifestyle can help you take a step forward in the right direction and even give you advice on what you do right and wrong and how to do it better. Reading gives you a stimulating control that helps you meet deadlines.

4.   Be creative

Sometimes only food can be the main motivation. Find a way to create what you want by using a shopping list or refrigerated content. You will find that following a vegetable diet is not difficult. Guess what? This is how you get results, pride and satisfaction (I have a recipe department in this book, so keep reading).

5.   Use the online support group

Always remember that you are not alone here, someone else found out what you know and survives. Although your friends and family do not support you, there are hundreds of online lifestyle groups where their members share stories, battles, recipes, and articles that can help you a lot.

Remember you can drop off the car in the beginning, but don't leave the car, do it and come back.

Is Vegetable Diet Expensive?

Did you know that you can eat a high-vegetables and all-products diet for about $ 3 a day? Yes, you read it correctly. I'm not talking about all the daily meals; I'm talking about **DAY** food, which is comparable to other meals. It is much less than the cost of food, whether it is cooked at home or elsewhere.

Not only does it control the quality of the foods it consumes, it also tastes tastier and healthier meals and spends about a third of what it would initially use for its meals.

vegetable diet

Designing nutritionally balanced vegetarian foods is not as difficult as it looks. It is known that some essential nutrients are linked to animal feeds, such as protein and iron, and a lack of knowledge about vegetarian foods that may provide or stop some people from changing their diet.

If you eat a variety of wholesome s plant products, you will get most of the terveellisist s nutrients, including protein, vitamins and minerals, such as iron and calcium. The only missing a lack of plant food nutrients are vitamin D and B vitamin which can easily get the supplements.

A healthy plant diet requires some awareness and knowledge, but once you've mastered the basics, you can quickly and easily make healthy, balanced meals every day. Feel this great strength as you understand how to eat properly and how to listen to your body's comments.

The first chapter looks at the key role of plants in maintaining health and weight. Let's now look at what a vegetarian diet looks like.

What is this?

Let's look at exactly what each term means.

Vegetarians do not eat animal meat (beef, fish, chicken, pork, lamb, etc.) and cannot use products that cause the death of the animal (such as skin).

Vegans do not eat animal products (vegetarian diet except dairy products, eggs, jellies or honey) and do not use products that cause animal death, cruelty or suffering (such as skin, wool or other existing products that have been tested on animals).) where possible and practical.

For proponents of **herbal** products, focus on whole plants and adopt healthy lifestyles to avoid highly refined foods and refined oils and highly refined, refined and cared for AZ.

Pescatariens eat fish but have no other **animal meat** , lots of dairy products, or eggs.

Flexitarians mainly eat vegetarians but are flexible in social situations.

The fact that motivation is primarily about the environment, ethics, or health can determine everyone's choices about what they buy and eat. Personally, I'm a vegan. I am motivated by three motivating factors of the vegan trifecta and focus on whole foods.

But the key is to research and focus on how to enjoy a wide variety of nutritious foods and eat a large portion of the diet, such as fresh fruits and vegetables, and I can make this flavor phenomenal, so I will never lose

DO NOT store the taste

Some people think that a plant-based diet consists of eating salads rather than eating the rest of their lives. If you are afraid or guilty of a diet based solely on your personal health, it is very difficult to maintain it for a long time, especially if the food is boring. Many clients come to me trying to use plants, but they are so tired of the food that they need help to maintain balance for a long time.

While I do not consider oils and sugars as healthy foods, it is a common benefit if they are used wisely to enhance taste and promote healthy eating in the long run. If a pinch of salt makes people eat more carrots, if the bank produces oil, they want people to eat more pumpkins for a profit. I wish this I would like a lot of attention after the lack of health and taste in bed, because they work very well together. In addition, the motivation to improve their health can go hand in hand by improving the health of our planet and reducing animal suffering. It turns out that Trifecta can help boost your motivation, which makes it truly a lifestyle, not a diet.

At first glance, people often think that herbal diets are extreme and restrictive. The truth is that now that wi ê more variety of product on the bed that yel these colors, look at the following desired six after information on the products food desired foods, vegetables, fruits, seeds and spices, and yel these sounds are never ± agricultural Coles, kt yellow Again the mind hears its cooks and it's much nicer! I never feel restricted or private; rather, it began in an exciting and tasty new world full of alternatives. May I introduce you to the rich world of the plant world you have found.

Vegetables are the starting point; They are so important that they should make up the majority of the diet. They include all the leaves, roots, bulbs, stems, vines and flowers listed here. Vegetables can be eaten in large quantities because most of them are water and fiber. They are full of vitamins and minerals and are an important source of potassium. Potassium is a mineral in the right proportion. Sodium regulates blood pressure. Sufficient potassium is just as important for people with high blood pressure as it is for reducing sodium intake.

foliage

One of the richest nutrients you can eat is green leafy vegetables. They contain many vitamins (especially K, A, C and folic acid) and minerals (such as iron, magnesium and potassium) and a large amount of chlorophyll, which purifies the human system, especially the liver. . If you're tired of salads, try adding vegetables to a cocktail or fruit soup. Vegetable puree is significantly reduced. It contains a wide variety of leaves of lettuce, cabbage, spinach, cabbage, swiss chard, meat, lettuce rocket like. Chinese cabbage, cabbage, green, mustard, dandelion, escarole, watercress, salt grass and tats.

roots

Root cultures usually consist of complex carbohydrates and starch. Therefore, they are usually boiled before eating, since boiling disintegrates the starch particles more easily. However, carrots and radishes are widely eaten raw in North America. Many tubers include carrots, beets, parsnips, fish marble, turnips, sweet potatoes, celery and radish. Many tubers, such as beets, radishes and turnips, also have leaves. delicious

light bulbs

This group includes onions, leeks and garlic. Strengthening the reputation of garlic affects the cardiovascular system. Many studies have shown that it lowers cholesterol, prevents platelet aggregation (when platelets bind, forms blood clots) and lowers blood pressure. Onion is also recommended. cardiovascular verisuoniterveyteen, because they have sulfur compounds that are the same as those that make s t garlic so strong.

rods

Stalk vegetables include asparagus, celery and cafe. These are very nutritious green vegetables with very few calories. Kohlrabi is a relative of cabbage and broccoli, and therefore it contains the vegetable family of potent anti-inflammatory and anti-cancer Connect days .

Live-Cam

Although some of these vegetables are considered to be fruitful in terms of nutrition and cooking, they fall into the category of vegetables. These vegetables have a high water content and are significantly reduced when cooked. Because of the variety of vegetables in this class, their nutritional profiles are very different, but the vines tend to be high in carotenoids and vitamin C. The vine plants are zucchini, pumpkin, eggplant, cucumber, peas, foil, tomato and pepper.

flower

Yes, flowers can also be vegetables! This group includes broccoli, cauliflower and artichokes. Broccoli, like dark green vegetables, is rich in nutrients and antioxidants. While the cauliflower is colorless, with similar nutrients and it is a total s good days for you than broccoli

mushrooms

Mushrooms are not really plants (they are mushrooms), but nutritionally they are combined with vegetables. The difference with fungi is that they eat organic matter and do not use photosynthesis like plants because they are a completely different organism than other vegetables. They are valuable in our diet because they provide a variety of nutrients, such as selenium ä and copper, as well s strongly inflammatory compounds, for protection against heart disease, cancer, protect and support the immune system. Fungi are rich in minerals and protein calories and are also a good source of B vitamins.

Some mushrooms found in the local market include chanterelles, shiitake, oysters, cremini, buttons, nest and balloons. There are many other edible fungi, including those used in Chinese medicine because of their medicinal properties. Some of them are strong enough to fight cancer.

fruit

Like vegetables, fruits are high in water and fiber, and rich in vitamins and minerals. Fruits are an important source of fast energy because they are broken down and used by the body, the fastest of all food groups . Fruits contain strong antioxidants, and because they are sweet, they are often more pleasant than vegetables, especially for children.

Wood fruits are available in summer and autumn and include apples, pears, plums and peaches. Citrus fruits are best in winter and include oranges, grapefruit, lemons and limes. Pure citrus juice can be used to flavor many herb recipes, including vegetables. Summer fruits are berries, grapes and melons. Tropical fruits include bananas, pineapples, mangoes and kiwi fruit.

Nuts and seeds

Nuts and seeds are a great source of strong nutrients, especially minerals, and contain healthy fats that help the body absorb and fully utilize these minerals. Studies have consistently shown that people who eat nuts have a lower risk of cardiovascular disease than those who do not. eating nuts is good that there are many types of nuts and seeds, because they all have different nutrients. Almonds, saksanp s nut s t, pistachios, cashews, walnuts, pumpkin seeds, sesame and flax seed are popular.

vegetables

Leguminous plants are leguminous plants; We usually eat fruits or seeds. They are an important source of lysine amino acid, high in fiber, vitamins and minerals and low in fat. They are healthier proteins than animal products, as well as cheaper protein per gram of protein. The best known legumes are peas, beans, lentils, peanuts and alfalfa.

Whole grains

Whole grains contain complex carbohydrates for energy sustaining s pit s order and are, in fiber, protein, vitamins (especially B vitamins A and E), minerals s LTT s m s tt o source systems of fatty acids and antioxidants. They are very difficult to digest, so they are usually cooked. the outer shells, while others have a shell with soft grains inside . Always choose whole grains where all the nutrients are intact instead of white, refined or polished grains that remain only in the starch cells. Currently, there are available a wide variety of whole jyvi s , with a variety of structures and flavors. N ä it s are rice, millet, buckwheat, oats, quinoa, spelled, barley and amaranth.

Spices and herbs

Spices and herbs are not only a way to add rich flavor to foods, but also contain small amounts of important nutrients. A study of Indian diet vegetarians found that they get 39-79% of the essential amino acids, as well as about 6% of calcium and 4% of iron, only in food spices.

Many spices contain protein, and although they contain too many grams, they are a source of some amino acids that may be low in vegetarian foods. Popular spices that give the world a taste are cumin, coriander, cinnamon, paprika and nutmeg.

Herbs such as parsley, coriander, mint, ginger and basil contain many nutrients and are most useful and tasty when freshly fed. Parsley gives women 22% of their daily vitamin C recommendations, and men 27% daily with only 4 tablespoons. All fresh herbs, such as green leafy vegetables, are rich in antioxidants and chlorophyll, which provide energy and help the body neutralize free radicals.

Nutrients in vegetarian foods

Food consists of macroelements (carbohydrates, fats and proteins) and micro-elements (vitamins and minerals) mixture . Carbohydrates should be the most important part of your daily intake. Fats are the second largest component followed by proteins, since fats provide twice the energy for the same volume, whereas when measuring portion sizes, fats and proteins should be almost equal.

Most people should try to eat 60-70% carbohydrates, 20-30% fat and 10-15% protein in the diet, and up to 20% protein for athletes is light. If your energy consumption is about 1500 calories, which I think is my average customer, it is between 225-263 grams of carbohydrates, 33-50 grams of fat and 38-56 grams of protein per day. The percentage you specify may be at the beginning or end of these areas, but these areas are suitable for about 98% of the population. Your position may vary slightly in life and season so listen to your body. Despite popular diet guides, you are unlikely to leave these beaches to no avail. Even older bodybuilders will never need more than 20% protein and can be harmful to the kidneys and metabolism in general.

If you are like most people, do not treat foods like carbohydrates or fats but rice or avocado. The advantage of plant -based foods is that they are much more nutritionally balanced than foods of animal origin. , which makes it easier to stay within the above normal limits without having to watch carefully what you eat. Consider the role of whole plant macronutrients in food.

carbohydrates

Some people are concerned about eating too much carbohydrate while eating vegetarian food. Carbohydrates are the body's most important source of energy and are perfectly healthy when used as whole grains (such as whole grains, vegetables, and fruits) because they contain many vitamins and minerals. , antioxidants, water and fiber. Fiber is also a carbohydrate, but its function is to aid digestion rather than provide energy.

Whole grains and fruits have the highest carbohydrate content, with a carbohydrate content of 70-90%. Eating a banana is an immediate boost of energy. The best sources of fiber in your diet are psyllium or flaxseeds and green leafy vegetables.

protein

It's not as difficult as people think about getting enough protein from vegetarian foods. All vegetarian foods contain protein. If you are consuming enough calories from a varied and balanced diet and are regular legumes, then proteins should eat more than enough and all the essential amino acids (which are the basic constituents of the protein). It is not necessary to combine several meals with a meal. get all the essential amino acids, which is a common mistake.

If the input range of products includes 48-hour days ll days , amino acids matingly s s ty o to perform.

Leguminous plants, including beans, have the highest total protein content in vegetable foods, about 18 to 25 percent; They are also important in vegetarian diets because they provide enough lysine amino acids. Green leafy vegetables have a high percentage of protein - 40 percent, spices add a small but significant amount of amino acids, and whole grains contribute a good amount of protein to a balanced diet, usually 8-12 percent. .

fat

Your body needs enough dietary fat to function, maintain its metabolism, and absorb and utilize minerals and some vitamins. People with cold feet and hands, menstruation (loss of menstruation), or dry skin, hair, or throat may need more fat in their diets, especially saturated fats such as coconut oil. obesity

Whole vegetarian foods are the best source of healthy fats: avocados, nuts and seeds (including peanut butter and seeds) On average, about 80% fat. Whole grains and beans also contain healthy fats and even fruits, vegetables, spices and almost all food products. They are even small, for example oatmeal contains 15% fat.

Oils are 100% fat, and you do not necessarily have to eat them, but they are excellent rich taste and t s perfected the taste on your plate, especially if you follow a healthier HCl diet. If k s co s s o ljyj days , it is best to keep HCl they minimize miss HCl and k s users HCl unpurified o ljyj days , such as olives, kookosp s hkinää, sesame, avocado (purified oils include rapeseed, soybean, sunflower and corn oils). You can fry vegetables easily with a teaspoon of oil.

However, this does not mean that you should never eat oils, and some people may benefit from concentrated fats. For example, flaxseed oil or concentrated DHA may be necessary for people with digestive problems who use omega-3 fatty acids.

This time I was training new students on the differences between a plant based diet and a vegan diet. I started by saying: "If you think , that a vegan and vegan diets are the same, raise your hand." It happened as I expected: 90% of the class raised their hands.

Vegetarian and vegan diets are really different. Like a plant-based diet, it's a lifestyle, just like veganism.

The vegan diet seriously rejects all kinds of animal products such as eggs, birds, honey, dairy products and even eyebrows in animal clothing. Vegans oppose striped skin or pet clothing, skin or use animals to test products. I noticed protests at fashion shows.

The goal of a vegetarian diet is to ensure that the food you eat is healthy, nutritious and beneficial to the body. This requires a lot of discipline, and this diet replaces plants with almost anything you can imagine in any animal feed.

Everything you eat in a plant-based diet serves a healthy diet. Up to 90% of Americans do not get the recommended daily harvest of fruit and vegetables; If you choose a herbal diet, you can be assured that you will get all the necessary and balanced nutrients that your body deserves.

Diets are similar, but vegetarian foods consume more plant and plant proteins, which reduces (or completely eliminates some animal products) animal products. There are people who follow a plant-based diet, eat meat, and there are people who follow or consume animal products.

A vegan diet, especially if you think about it, can be healthy, but a herbal diet has more benefits than a vegan diet because it consists of avoiding fully processed foods and sticking to all foods. They are densely nutritious, as all vegans have described; A good example is vegan cookies or vegan ice cream.

Thanks to herbal diet, it reduces the risk of heart disease and other diseases. This is one of the best ways to strengthen the immune system by supporting the body's metabolism . It's also a great way to start your journey to slimming.

Vegetable: The diet is also known as any food or vegetable, it is as simple as it sounds. It is a diet that has been developed with or without meals, all foods (for example, all natural, raw or unrefined) and herbal (farmed or plant based) foods.

At the moment, I can say devotion simply by changing our eating habits and lifestyle, eating refined foods, processed and stored, when you grow food on farms or plants and some animal products (in some cases).

Herbal meals consist of

Vegetables: such as lettuce, cabbage, Swiss turkey, pepper, peas, sweet corn, etc.

Cereals: millet, quinoa, barley, rice, wheat, oats, etc.

Tubers: sweet potatoes, potatoes, sweet potatoes, carrots, beets, etc.

Legumes: beans, chick peas, cannellini beans, lentils, black beans, etc.

Seeds: such as sorghum, chia seeds, sesame seeds, etc.

Fruits: such as apples, bananas, figs, grapes, strawberries, oranges, etc.

It seems to me that s for many people who do not understand what it is food or plant life;

Vegan Diet: This is a completely vegetarian diet that excludes meat, fish, dairy and eggs. In essence, it excludes any food of animal or animal origin.

Vegetarian Diet: This is also a vegetarian diet but includes animal products such as diary and eggs in meal planning.

Flexographic Diet: This is a vegetarian diet that allows meat and fish but is still a vegetarian diet.

Fish-based diet: This is also a vegetable-based diet that includes eggs, program, fish and shellfish, but meat and poultry are not included.

Plant-based diets are sometimes blended with a vegetarian diet or a vegan diet simply because, unlike a vegetarian diet, this product does not completely eliminate animal products. This diet simply chooses many vegetarian foods.

It depends mainly on vegetables, fruits, seeds, legumes, nuts and whole grains as they make up the majority of the meals.

While there are many types of vegetarian diets and all claiming to be associated with cardiac benefits (such as whole grains, fruits, vegetables, legumes, nuts, and healthy oils) high in fiber, vitamins and minerals that lower blood pressure and LDL, the risk of diabetes helps maintain your health. one must always consider the types of herbal foods and their sources.

A healthy vegetable meal should consist of appropriate portions of vegetables, whole grains, fruits and proteins, healthy and healthy oils.

A plant-based diet or lifestyle is quite easy and flexible because it consumes more plants even if animal products are not fully available.

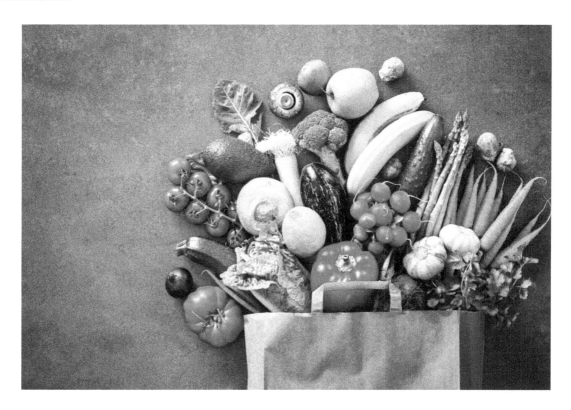

10 PLANT CONTROL

There is so much fashionable food in today's news. They are fun because they are new and exotic. You may be surprised to find that many of the products you see daily are rich in nutrients. We give these superheroes every day. They deserve recognition.

1. Parsley

• High iron content used by the body to generate energy and transport oxygen.

• Rich in vitamin C, which stimulates the immune system and supports iron absorption.

• Extremely rich in Vitamin K, which is part of a healthy bone structure, prevents blood clots and keeps nails strong.

• Rich in vitamin A, which maintains eye function, maintains the immune system, and cleanses acne, rash and psoriasis.

2. Chia seeds

• One of the best sources of omega-3 fatty acids.

• Keep the mix of soluble and insoluble fiber gut health in order to maintain.

• High in calcium, which helps maintain bones, minimizes muscle spasms and helps you sleep.

3. Cinema, amaranth and teff

• High in protein, good for beans if it produces gas.

• Higher levels of quercetin and kaempferol than other foods. These two compounds help to reduce the inflammatory response to allergens.

• A good source of manganese (which promotes healthy bones, skin and blood sugar), magnesium, folic acid (which helps maintain a healthy brain, cardiovascular system and pregnancy), zinc and vitamin E.

4. buckwheat

• A good source of routine, a vegetable pigment that can prevent blood clots, thyroid problems, memory loss, osteoarthritis and varicose veins.

• High vitamin B content for energy and fat metabolism.

• High levels of antioxidants to combat free radicals caused by aging, cancer, atherosclerosis and other problems.

• Contains a compound called D-Chiro-inositol which helps to balance blood sugar.

5. berries

• An extremely rich source of antioxidants (which become organic or wild in overdose) that prevent cell damage, and berries are found to be particularly useful in maintaining memory.

• Low glycemic index (40-50; less than 50 indicates low), as studies show improved glycemic control.

• High levels of manganese to help maintain healthy bones and skin and balance blood sugar levels.

• Some women swear that they help to reduce hot flashes.

6. Pumpkin

• Rich in Vitamin A, which supports the health of the eyes, skin and immune system.

• High levels of all carotenoids (bright red, yellow and orange responsible for plant pigments), including alpha, beta, lutein, zeaxanthin and beta-cryptoxanthines, which are antioxidants and have anti-inflammatory and immunological properties.

• Starch comes from a polysaccharide containing special compounds called homogalacturonan, which have antioxidant, anti-inflammatory, diabetic and insulin-regulating properties.

7. Avocados

• High level of potassium in the sodium to achieve healthy blood pressure.

• Contains healthy fats that help the body absorb vitamins A, D, and E, K and minerals. Avocado fat is mostly monounsaturated, which has been shown to reduce the risk of heart lowering LDL cholesterol (the bad type) and reducing the amount of oxidative stress in the blood.

• A good source of B vitamins, A and K.

8. Chickpeas

• High in manganese, folic acid, iron and zinc.

• Complex carbohydrates for energy and a protein source that assists muscles, digestion, hormones, neurotransmitters, genomes, blood pressure, energy and detoxification.

• contains a different type of fiber, which leads to better control of blood lipids, lowering LDL cholesterol, total cholesterol, triglycerides, blood glucose and insulin secretion, and colon bacteria metabolize it to produce compounds that act vuorauspolttoaineena intestinal cell walls. , which reduces the risk of colorectal cancer.

9. Brazil nuts and sunflower seeds

• High level of zinc, which helps strengthen the immune system and maintain healthy skin and the male genitalia.

• A good source of selenium that supports the immune system, detoxifies the liver, supports the function of the thyroid gland, prevents certain cancers and maintains healthy hair, skin and nails.

• Rich in vitamin E, an antioxidant that helps protect the cardiovascular system.

10 ginger

• Supports digestion, increases metabolism; It has anti-inflammatory and immunostimulatory effects.

• Ginger You were able to inhibit colon cancer cell growth and cause cell death in ovarian cancer cells.

Nutrition tips to stay strong and focused

As a Holistic Nutrition Therapist, I think you should go for a healthy lifestyle if you want to grow and find the energy and health you are looking for. This path includes what you eat, what you don't eat, what you do during the day, and especially the attitude that is brought to the table.

But I don't think I have to do it all at the same time. And I really don't think it's perfect. I have a live test, such as hundreds of customers. I worked on a step-by-step, external approach to changing my diet, which can work wonders. The most important thing is to get started. Focus on the cooking you love daily and celebrate your success. Here are tips and motives to stay strong on this path.

Remove meat and seafood

Replaces burgers for vegetarians. The meat contains an inflammatory compound called arachidonic acid as well as saturated fat and cholesterol. Cows produce 150 billion liters of methane a day, which contributes significantly to global warming. One pound of meat requires 2500 liters of water. .

Remove dairy products and eggs.

Replace dairy products with almond milk and coconut yoghurt and non-dairy products. Dairy products are one of the most common factors that cause food intolerance and the cause of common acne. One kilogram of cheese requires 900 liters of water. A gallon of milk requires 1000 liters of water.

Replace the eggs with flax or chia seeds. Or try this mix in Chapter 7. To produce a kilo of eggs you need 477 liters of water. Although the health of eggs is being discussed, they do not add nutrients that we were unable to produce. "They have not been found elsewhere, and diabetics can increase the risk of heart disease.

Avoid processed and refined foods.

Processed foods are those that have changed shape. Every time we cook or pass, we deal with it. Human sauces and butter beans are healthy processed foods because they still contain all the natural nutrients.

Sophisticated products are those that have removed these parts and also the most important parts of the diet. White flour and white sugar are refined, as are white rice and oils such as rapeseed. When food is processed, it loses fiber, proteins, vitamins and minerals. After cleaning, the remainder of the grain is mainly starch, which contains small amounts of some nutrients. Therefore, they are called empty calories. They help your body always need nutrients, but they increase calories a day.

Focus on whole foods

All products are as close as possible to their natural shape. Fresh vegetables, fruits, whole grains, beans and pulses, nuts and seeds are healthy products. By consuming all products, you maximize the nutrient density of all vitamins and minerals. and antioxidants in these products. It also reduces calorie density, as these products are high in fiber and water, so they fill you up without extra calories.

Chew the food

Not only does it slow down a bit of an enjoyable meal, you can also feel it easier when full, but it is also the first important step in digestion without Sufficient chewing of carbohydrates does not completely drop and can later cause gas or indigestion.

Avoid high doses

Usually, the dishes at the restaurant are much more than what you need to eat (unless you are in the eye of a stylish restaurant). Get in touch with the right parts by trying out the recipes and meals in this book . The recipes speak of the number of servings. Take these numbers seriously, divide the dishes and see what it feels like to eat a normal sized serving. Chew slowly and begin to control your hunger and satiety. This is the best way to find out how much you need to feed, but don't overeat your body.

Hey eat

Most nutrition tips and healthy meals are boring. Have fun and enjoy your taste buds with a fun meal. Yes, he can still be healthy. Try one of the pizza or vegetable hamburger recipes in this book, or have a Mexican evening with burritos, tacos or fajitas for cooking.

Take supplements

These Vitamin B supplements are essential, they are completely herbal, and adults over 50, regardless of their diet, as well as those who suffer from digestive problems. If anyone suggests eating eggs or other animal products as the best or most natural way to get vitamin B , remember that animals do not produce vitamin B ; It is produced by bacteria in the digestion of animals. Elderly and ruoansulatushäiriöiset people can not get B12 from food, so supplements are the most effective way to get a B12

In the United States, the recommended daily allowance (RDA) for vitamin B is 24 micrograms per day for most adults and 28 micrograms for pregnant or breast-feeding women. Newer research increases the ideal yield by 4-7 micrograms per day. Vitamins B stimulate energy and the nervous system, so it is best to take them in the morning and early afternoon so they do not merge before going to bed.

Without vitamin D you will not be able to absorb and use calcium properly. Deficiency of calcium and vitamin D weakens bones. Researchers have also begun to link vitamin D deficiency to all health problems and illnesses, including asthma and cancer. Carnivores should also take care of this. According to a 2009 study, most vegetarians (59 percent) and those eating meat (64 percent) do not have enough vitamin D.

Vegetarian foods do not contain vitamin D, but our bodies naturally produce it when our skin is exposed to the sun. However, it is difficult to measure and count, because we produce a variety of m HCl ri s skin v s rist s and other factor ö ist s , depending, in winter, there is usually not as much sunlight as in summer. The more northern the more winter affects vitamin D levels, and if it is far north, you may not get it in winter. The recommended daily dose is 600 IU a day, but for optimal health, supplementing between 1,000 and 2,000 IU a day has proven to be good for most people. Up to 4000 IU is safe for most adults.

The cause of calcium deficiency is not always low intake, and vegetable sources are often a better option than dairy products because they contain magnesium, which helps in mineral absorption. Because calcium is such an important nutrient, it is difficult to get enough food without consuming too many calories. The average food intake is about 700 mg per day and the recommended dose for adults is 1000 mg (up to 1300 mg for the elderly). This means that an add-on that allows you to increase these 300mg more may be helpful.

Our body also needs two special fatty acids from our diet: omega-3 and omega-6. Others can occur in our bodies if we usually eat enough fat. The difficulty is that our body needs a certain amount of omega-3 to omega-6 fatty acids. Most dietary sources contain too much omega-6 fatty acids, which results in a relative lack of omega-3 fatty acids. The strongest dietary sources of omega-3 fatty acids are ground flaxseeds, flaxseed oil, chia seeds and sachainchi oil, and amazon oil. The ground flaxseeds are large but can be difficult to digest and absorb. If you want to get enough omega-3 fatty acids, oils   Linen, Chia and sachainchi (also known as Inca nuts) are great ways to do this.

There is a special type of omega-3 called DHA that is important for brain and nerve function. Your body converts omega-3 to DHA, but it's not always effective. Taking DHA 200-300 mg is often the best way to get this nutrient. People who need more long-chain n-3, such as women in pregnancy and breastfeeding, children and people with digestive or nervous problems , benefit from supplementing DHA with plenty.

Digestive enzyme supplements and / or probiotics may be helpful when switching to a vegetarian diet if you have problems digesting beans. Incomplete digestion is one of the major causes of nutritional deficiencies, as well as food allergies and intolerances. They need antibiotics after probiotics to colonize a healthy intestinal flora.

FOODS

To succeed and take responsibility, you need to model the environment according to your goals, starting with what is brought to the kitchen and putting it on your body. If you make sure your kitchen is full of healthy foods, you can always prepare a well-balanced meal. Although you do not have exactly what a particular recipe needs, you will need ingredients that you need to replace. Let's change our kitchen.

Food Storage

We add flour, sugars, and refined oils, and choose healthy, unrefined versions. Serve us with whole grains, beans, legumes and nuts.

• Whole grains (brown rice, quinoa, buckwheat, millet).

• Beans and legumes (chick peas, beans, lentils).

• Nuts (raisins, dates, dried apricots, berries).

• crude oils (olives, coconuts, roasted sesame seeds)

• Vinegar (apple, balsamic, wine).

• Wholemeal flour (whole grains, spelled, oats, buckwheat).

• Unsweetened sweeteners (raw cane sugar such as succinate, coconut sugar, maple syrup, molasses, pure stevia).

• sea salt.

• Spices (ginger, cumin, coriander, turmeric, pepper, cinnamon).

• Dried herbs (basil, oregano, thyme, dill, mixed herbs).

• yeast.

fridge

We put meat, cheese, milk, eggs and packaged food. We supply fresh products, nuts and seeds and other dairy products.

• Green leaves (lettuce, cabbage, Swiss mainland, spinach).

• Fresh herbs and spices (parsley, basil, mint, garlic, ginger).

• Green / starchy vegetables (cucumber, pepper, green beans, broccoli, mushrooms).

• Starchy vegetables (carrots, beets, sweet potatoes, winter pumpkin)

• Onions (sweet, red, yellow, green).

• Fruits (apples, oranges, plums, grapes, melons).

• Nuts and seeds (almonds, nuts, sunflower seeds, chia seeds, flax seeds).

• Peanut Butter and Seeds (Peanuts, Almonds, Fish Nuts, Sunflower)

• Non-milk milk (almonds, soybeans).

freezer

Time to get rid of TV dinners, potatoes, frozen waffles, ice cream, cakes and frozen desserts. Store fresh frozen and homemade products.

• Frozen berries, mangoes, melon.

- Ripe frozen banana smoothies and cream sorbets.
- Edamame beans, peas, sweet corn, broccoli, spinach and other frozen whole vegetables.
- Highly cooked and frozen in individual batches (soups, stews, peppers, tomato sauce, vegetable burgers)
- Healthy confectionery (cakes, cups, pies, fruit cakes).

Home fast food factory

Sometimes we don't have time to follow the rules. I have now created a draft of a balanced aterista, so you can connect it to the kitchen.

mixer

Prepare a perfect nutritious cocktail to start the day and feed it. You will need:

- Glass and straw: Reusable straws minimize contact with your teeth for better dental health, and the use of an insulated cup or travel mug makes a cocktail known in the morning.
- Creamy: bananas (frozen computer brands such as ice cream), avocados, peanut butter or milk without milk.
- Omega-3: 1 tablespoon of flax or chia seeds.

Protein: a handful of oatmeal or quinoa or a tablespoon of vegetable protein powder.

- Fruit: about 1 cup blueberry, watermelon, grapes, apples L paths of any shape.

• Fortify vegetables: vegetables such as spinach, sprouts or cabbage; vegetables such as cucumbers or carrots; Fresh herbs such as mint or basil.

• Rise of food baskets: fresh ginger, powdered green leaves, matcha powder, probiotics, berries or goji powder, cocoa beans.

bowl

Build the perfect bowl for lunch or dinner that will provide you with all the nutrients and fuel you need for the rest of the day. You will need:

Bowl: Get a pair of the same size to hold the same portions

• Green leafy vegetables: Take a handful or two as much as you want, lettuce, cheeseburger, spinach, cabbage, Swiss lime, parsley or other vegetables.

• Starchy vegetables and / or whole grains: About 1 cup sweet potatoes, winter pumpkin, brown rice, quinoa, spelled, Soba noodles, rice noodles, etc.

• Beans or legumes: about ½ cup beans, black beans, lentils, edamame or other legumes.

• Other vegetables: about 1 cup of raw vegetables such as cucumber, pepper, tomato and avocado; grilled such as zucchini, eggplant and mushrooms; or steamed like broccoli, carrot and beetroot.

• Nuts or seeds: a small handful (pumpkin, cashew, almonds) or peanut butter that can be used as a base for sauce.

• Sauce: long and rich fillet. Try the recipes in this book, such as sesame and baked misokastiketta, jumalatarikastiketta green or creamy balsamikastiketta, or check the ingredients, you can store a variety of dishes.

GROUPS OF FOODS

We all know that herbal diets are important for our well-being and health, especially when it comes to preventing heart disease. However, as Fred's father experienced, researchers have said that there are herbal diets that can be harmful to health. Health of your heart.

According to the United States Center for Disease Control (CDC), six hundred thousand people die each year from heart disease. The main cause of this death has been identified as poor nutrition, which is the driving force behind heart disease.

Much research has been done to show the many benefits of whole grains, vegetables, legumes, flaxseeds, and fruits; These products have been identified as the right type of diet to end coronary heart disease.

Another analysis showed that the diet contains vegetables, the best kind of desired feeding for humans and ± diseases ê ischemic ± heart.

According to the latest comprehensive study on the benefits and risks of a herbal diet. The study was conducted on approximately 209,289 persons, including 43,259 men and 166,030 women, according to nurses and health care professionals. The study took about 20 years to understand participants' lifestyles, health behaviors, and medical history. Participants in this study have never had a stroke, cancer, coronary or coronary surgery. About 8,631 patients with coronary artery disease were followed up.

One of the main reasons for these studies is the difference between diets: vegetarian and vegetarian diets. He intended to distinguish between different types of vegetarian based on the pros and cons.

The researchers decided to focus on diets and developed three different diets:

Vegetarian diet consisting of foods derived from unhealthy plants. These include refined cereals, sweet drinks, sweets and potatoes.

Vegetarian foods that use vegetarian foods and allow foods that contain animals or nutrients.

Herbal products that focus on healthy foods of plant origin: whole grains, vegetables, fruits, legumes (these products are more organic).

FOOD DESIGN BUILDING GUIDE

Buy fresh

Buy products as fresh as possible, cultivated locally and organically whenever possible. Expand yours if possible. Sprouts and herbs can easily be grown on a windowsill. If you use the pantry entire jyvi s and spices, replace the old after about a year. If you start with fresh, high quality ingredients, meals will naturally taste better.

Select the products you want

Choose most vegetables and other better products. Get diversity by introducing new ones from time to time, but this is not always the case. Some products are naturally tastier than others for most people. The natural sweetness of pumpkins, sweet potatoes, peppers, carrots and beets makes them more attractive. Vegetables and legumes are often softer and sweeter than their fully developed counterparts.

Choose cooking methods

Use the correct cooking method. Avocados are raw, broccoli is cooked to a bit of perfection (but it becomes bitter if cooked), sweet potatoes and squash are delicious in the oven or in the oven. Whole grains are cooked at different times and can be pre-cooked to improve flavor.

Find good combinations

The meal combination of the dish consists of a combination of aromas (sweet, salty, sour) and textures (crisp, sweet). Color also plays an important role in making the vase more visually appealing. He wants to combine opposites (bitter) or similarities (all greens). These are also personal preference s , so try the recipes data ä and then play combinations to see what you like.

Use salt

A small amount of salt has a great influence on the taste of the food, reducing the bitterness of the vegetables and their consistency. It helps to destroy the walls of plant cells, which facilitates their melting from production.   . It allows you to combine all food flavors so that hummus does not know the individual ingredients but hummus. When cooking, use salt, rub it to moisten vegetables before cooking, or sprinkle with lightly salted sauce in a bowl or salad.

Season the beans

Beans and beans do not taste good Make them more interesting by:

• Combine with fresh and tasty fruits or vegetables.

• Add spices, herbs or tea while boiling in water.

• Use some or all of the vegetable broth or juice for cooking.

• Season with spices and salty sauces.

cordially

Each dish can be delicious with the right spice or sauce. Chopped vegetables in a good sauce soften the bitterness and texture and help to combine the flavors of the vegetables and the sauce. Marinate the beans and all the beans in the sauce for an hour (or day) to saturate so that they are full of flavor.

Add dessert

Use natural sweets in your kitchen. Try balm sauce, maple syrup or apple mousse; Add apples, oranges, dried cranberries or raisins to salad or soup.

Use healthy fats

Fat makes a dish richer and more rewarding. Fats taste spicy evening and yrtteiltä, so k s co ä them ä extremely s in tasty dishes. K s employee s more th s n fat vegetarian diet j days after that, or if you are not accustomed to healthy cooking. Try fats in most foods, such as p s nut ö sheets, seeds and avocado, instead of fats that are naturally part of boiled foods, exercise. A mixture of peanut butter and seeds or avocado is a great cream base for sauce or sauce.

camouflage

Be smart! Mix vegetables and vegetables in soups, sauces or cocktails. Bake vegetables with specialties like carrot cake , zucchini bread, pumpkin muffins, chocolate beetroot infusion and sweet potato cakes.

Live plans

Are you ready to increase the nutritional value, flavor and energy of your food? Anything can happen right away, I promise! I developed these meal plans to show you how to make delicious herbal foods that provide balanced nutrition and nutrition throughout the day.

Plans for the next three weeks will remove assumptions from the kitchen's vegetable diet. There are three meals a day and snack options to choose from in a matter of weeks. Chapter 3 contains more recipes than meal plans. This leaves room for flexibility, so if one of your meal plans is not satisfactory for you, switch to another recipe.

These meal plans use leftovers to make your life easier because most of us do not have the time to prepare three meals a day. Breakfast and lunch must be brought and picked up from Monday to Friday. I also give advice on how to prepare for the week so you can prepare for success.

Desserts aren't included in the plan, but you can try Chapter 11 desserts if you like, or if you're having a party or a meal you want to bring something you like.

Our goal is to be healthy, full of energy, content and happy until the end of this plan.

Sleep a little

Some studies show that sleep affects the part of the brain that controls willpower. Therefore, if you are awake, it is more difficult to resist temptation. His ability to make clear decisions is impaired, which increases the likelihood of eating that he does not eat. "I really need it.

Nor is it able to deal with stress in a constructive way, which makes it more susceptible to overeating or other negative compensation mechanisms. Regular, high quality sleep not only makes you healthier and more energetic, but also helps you manage your desires. Here are some ways to develop healthy sleeping habits.

• Try to have about the same time to wake up and sleep every day.

• Do not use your TV, computer, tablet or phone for 30 minutes before going to bed

• Do not exercise after lunch.

• Caffeine deficiency after 2 pM

• After lunch without sugar.

• Try meditation, restorative yoga or something relaxing at night.

Active three times a week.

Exercise is crucial for maintaining bone mass, cardiovascular health, lymphatic and immune systems, and can help prevent diabetes. Exercise also releases hormones in the blood that make you happy, reduce hunger and   Usually it maintains the proper functioning of the body. Try a quick workout after work, and it may not be such a great meal for dinner.

Regular exercise helps to reduce fatigue, depression, tension, anxiety and discomfort; Improve your mood and your ability to handle stressful situations. As you become stronger and have more resistance, your body will function more efficiently. Start with what you want: walking, roller skating, hula hula. If you like it, you are more likely to like it for a long time. semester. Show something you can do for 20-30 minutes three times a week. It doesn't always have to be the same mix to interest you. Once you get used to it, you can add new days, spend more time, or try something intense.

Don't insist on being perfect

Stress affects health and excessive food stress is harmful. It would be great if you could still eat a perfect diet and maintain an ideal exercise plan, but I don't know anyone who could do it daily. You will feel guilty if you have a day that is not ideal as it will only bring negative energy into your life. Some people eat more when they are not feeling well. I don't want to use the words "slip", "trap" or "bug" because. I believe that everything we do is just part of life and makes us the person we want. I know tomorrow

Don't punish yourself with less food or more exercise. Instead, write a letter every day and go further, revitalize, maintain or possibly adjust your plans for the future to work for you in real life.

Listen to your body and enjoy it!

Maintaining a balance does not always mean strict diet plans or rules; It means finding the right balance for your body's needs. Now that you are looking for better health, you can get back in touch and trust your gut to continue learning what works for you. Eat consciously, chew food well, taste and taste when you eat enough

With your body in balance and following the principles of a long-term healthy diet, you should be able to hear your body's messages about what should be healthy. Every person is different and has a different way of being healthy. However, your body's messages can be distorted or muted when they are unbalanced, so it is difficult to determine at first whether you think there is real desire or hunger.

Positive energy can have a big impact on your goals. It is unfortunate that many diet programs focus on avoiding unhealthy foods by switching to a healthy diet because it is much nicer and more effective to focus on eating good foods. such as fruits, nuts, or a special dinner, and eat them often to keep you happy and excited about a healthy lifestyle.

WEEKU VEGAN'S MANUFACTURING PLAN

week

CONTRACT NOTICE

Breakfast: vanilla, pudding 1 tablespoon fresh soda

Lunh: Fluffy Crisp and Open Water Low in Oil or Sweet Potato (Marinated)

Snorkel behind: 1/4 cups hemp powder with fresh vegetables (wrinkles, flowers, romaine salad, balls, etc.)

Dinner: Black beans and salad uinoa salad q uick cumin drosesing

DESSERT: Spider shock

Tuesday

Winds are as follows: Cocktail, 1 almond raisin, 1 tear, banana, 1, 2 times.

Lunch: 1 brown roasted coffee (for toast) or two gluten-free cakes with fresh or toasted 1/4 hummus tortilla are a bit strong. SEE FLOWERING EQUIPMENT WELCOME OR DURING.

After a snack: a protein bar

Lunch: Zuchini pasta with chryrry tomatoes, sweet potatoes, balsam and hemp.

DESSERT: BANANA SUPPORT

Wednesday

Best for: Fifth success as soon as possible with 1 tbsp fresh beans

Food: said at least three cups of green vegetables you would like to get 3 caps or treasures and one from Koszenocero.

Afternoon snack: 4 tablespoons of hummingbird with fresh vegetables (wrinkles, celery, lettuce, balls, etc.)

Dinner: Cappuccino, it's a date ddddd tru d tru d tru tru tru dd dddddddddddddddddddddddd

Dessert: 2 pieces of raw brownies

Thursday

Best for: Nirvana chillies and chocolate, fresh fruit is recommended

LUNH: I just made a salad with 1/2 cup of organic drink

Behind the snorkel: 1 ounce. Almonds and a few tablespoons of raisins

Lunch: Summer quiz and perfect spot (obtained from q or uinnaa paacra for brown)

PROJECT: 2 EXTREMELY EXCLUSIVE MASSAGES

Friday

More importantly, a smiling face with 1 cup of almonds, 1 cup of berries, 1 cup of nutritious chocolate chocolate, 3 tablespoons of salads and 1 cup of coffee milk.

€ 15.00

Snout: 2 options with almond butter

Dinner: Buttruther s ash curry serves the way cup cooked q uinoa, steamedeeeerables as desire d

Dessert: dark chocolates

Saturday

Breakfast: oatmeal and almond butter

Lunh: Smiley, avoid and say jícam

Snack back: 1 tablespoon of almonds mixed with nutritional protein powder and several cubes

DENNER: Burgers and Black Grains, Served with Small Salad or Steamed Vegetables

Dessert: 2 types of vanilla and vanilla

Sundays

Breakfast: small 1/2 ice cream, 1 cup ice, 2 ice cubes, 3/4 cups starch, 1 cup green leafy vegetables and 1 serving of nutritious vanilla.

Lunh: He left the previous burger and burger, he said.

Second snack: 1/4 cup vegan mix (or 2 tablespoons almond or pine nuts and 2 tablespoons dried fruit)

Dinner 1 cup of selected q uinoa, browned rice, or in the case of served Half chopped avocado 1 cup steamede greens and of chomo sauce.

Dessert: 1/2 cup chocolate

ALL WEEKS

On Monday,

Best for: gluten-free banana pancake, served with 1 cup of fresh beans

Lunch: Mango, Kale, and avassal d

Snack: Afternoon, bread, paddle, berrée or other selected fresh fruit.

DENNER: ROLLANTINATION OF EGG VEGETABLES EXAMPLES OF TRUCKS, GOODS OR BROKOLO

PROJECTS: DARKL SHOCK

Tuesday

Best for: Cinnamon

Lunch: pumpkin and apple soup, served with fresh green vegetables or selected carved vegetables

Afternoon snack: nutrition at the bar

Note: Raw zucchini is eaten with basil and various cakes, served with sauces or such stressful sausages.

PROJECT: 2 vegan cookies
Wednesday

Small addition: Cocktail 1 cut into bluish designs or blends containing 1 cup coconut and half water to be included in plan 1 chocolate according to cooking plan

Lunch: Easy to grow yellow lentil with avocado croutons

Snack: fresh vegetables, 1/4 cup hummus

Day: salad or black rice and amaranth with delicate cumin

DESIGN: 1/2 cups from the collection
Thursday

Most important: 1 bread bath, 1 cup of organic or delicious coffee (I like white bread) and 1 cup of almond milk

Lunch: apples, portions and crispy curry sauce

Previous answer: 1/4 cups of real powder mixture according to your choice

Dinner: SWETT POTATATE LIMMER BURBERERS, say first or say VEGETAL as he wanted

DESIGN: 2 raw vanilla noodles
Friday

Best: VANILLA butter pudding with 1 cup fresh soda

Lunch: The front, is outside, and said many rockets.

Afternoon: Group of walnuts and raw walnut jelly

Lunch: sweet potatoes and milk are made with broccoli or steamed vegetables

PROJECT: 1/2 Chocolate
Saturday

Breakfast: Smoothie with 1 frozen banana, 1/2 tablespoon fried mango, 1 tablespoon hippie, 1 cup avocado and 1/2 cup coconut.

Lunch: WHITE LOOP LORD AND USE CHILD OR GREEN GREEN

Afternoon snack: Nutrition instead of choice

Lunch: "Rice" with lemon, lemon and pistachios, served with fresh vegetables

PROJECT: DELIVERY OF RAW MILK

Sunday

Best: BANANA AND FEES

Lunch: An avocado carrot is a good buy for a salad.

Snorkel Back: Raw vegetables with sweet potato humus

Lunch: brown rice with lentils, served with fresh salad or steamed vegetables and for eating.

Dessert: 2 many misc
CONTINUE THREE
CONTRACT NOTICE

Best for: gia with stiff pudding with chia

Lunch: leftover brown rice and lentils, lots of mixed vegetables and many reception options.

Afternoon aperitif: 2 scoops of peanut butter and snacks

Note: Raw "nuts" are not consumed with steamed vegetables or at your discretion.

DESIGN: Dark chocolate
Teseas

Breakfast: cocktail with 1 glass of almonds, 1 large frozen bread, 1-2 tablespoons at a time, 1 serving of powder and cup filled with granules, lots and lots of grains.

Lunch: mango, avocado and avocado

Afternoon Snack: True Vegetarian and HUMMUS ANNUAL REPORT

Lunch: Easy rice without beans and vegetables

Dessert: 2 raw and vegan cookies
Wednesday

Breakfast: BANANAN BRAAKFASS WRAPS

Lunh: Omelette and fresh fish salad.

Snack: Restaurant Bar

Lunch: Arugulana with cooking and fruits, blueberries and tasty

PROJECT: Banana contains something else
Thursday

Best for: Cinnamon Apple

Lunch: fennel salad, avocado and tomatoes 1/2 tbsp white beans or white beans

Snack: 1 group of people mixed with protective powder

Lunch: It is said that most baked cakes are tinned.

Dessert: dark chocolates
Friday

Breakfast: gluten-free vegan muffins with a spoon of almond butter and a plate

Lunch: apples, portions and chrysanthemum; 1 cup rice and mushroom soup

Snack: 1/3 cup raw fruit mix (or a mix of almonds, raisins or jelly beans)

Lunch: some mustard is cut into large pieces and "weeping" and "weeping" steamed with boiled broccoli or broccoli.

PROJECT: Waffle ginger is creamy
Saturday

In a nutshell: SmOththie with 1 ½ cups of blue water or fruit mixture, 1 grape with nuts, 1/2 small amount of water, 1 high surface resistance.

Lunh: easily wrapped in "croutons", served with lots of sauces or steamed drinks.

After a snack: Officer sticks stored 2 tablespoons of nuts or almonds and raisins ("ants in logs")

Note: After a large amount of raw vegetables and selected vegetables, 1 cup cooked oysters, 1/2 ½ cup, ½ cup, ½ cup of coffee, ingredients and unique label sauce.

PROJECT: 2 rare, highly visible
Sunday

Key Features: 1 slice of banana and fresh fruit, rice, 1 cup or organic millet, full of rice (I like the Arrowhead Mills brand) and 1 cup of corn.

Lunch: smoked avocado and jicama, 1 small, if desired

Back snorkel: 2 balls of walnuts and Japanese cereal straight

Dinner: Quinnaencillas

Dessert: Sugar chocolate
Four weeks
CONTRACT NOTICE

Most importantly, cut 1 frozen banana, 1/2 frozen Mug, 1 canola, 1 tablespoon coconut and 1/2 cup wine

Lunch: leftover food in the kitchen, talking to selected salad dressing

Snack: Selected food bar

Lunch: Arugulá declared the roasted pumpkin, swallowed it, and fled.

PROJECT: 2 EXTREMELY EXCLUSIVE MASSAGES
Tuesday

Breakfast: Vánnila can hug one cup of fresh berries

Dinner: the red flame and finally the ragula said in good taste

Afternoon snack: lots of raw peanut butter and jelly beans

Dinner: The offer of sweets and black beans is made from broccoli or coarse.

Dessert: 1/2 cup chocolate
Wednesday

Best for: 1 cocktail of frozen bread, 1/2 tablespoon of frozen ice cream, 1 tablespoon of spinach leaves, 1 cup of avocado nuts and 1/2 cup of wine

Lunh: Boll with smaller black beans and sweet potatoes in large quantities.

Next dive: diet choice

Lunch: Cauliflower "water" with lemon, mint and beans stored in large quantities

Dessert: Serve chocolate with almonds
Thursday

Note: Smiling face with 1 tablespoon of almonds, 1 large frozen banana, 1-2 tablespoons at a time, 1 serving of protein powder and lots of creams (spinach, approx.

Lunch: 1 freshly made rice tortilla (for life) or oatmeal with 1/4 inch cocoa tortillas, roasted or roasted peppers and lots of green leaves. Serve if desired with steamed vegetables or in a small dish.

Diving Back: Basic Nutrition

DENNER: zucchini paste with tomato cake, sweet potato, basil and parmesan cheese

Dessert: soft banana
Friday

Most important: Apple introduces itself right away

Lunch: fried pumpkin and big soup, served with steamed or steamed vegetables

Afternoon snack: nutrition bar

DENNER: Raw ZuChin with Alfredo cherry and cherry tomato, served with fresh salads or vegetables of your choice.

PROJECT: 2 real brownie rats
Saturday

Best of all: smiling face 1 cup frozen or mixed berries, 1 cup walnut water, 1/2 small avocado, 1 serving chocolate and a pinch of porridge.

Lunch: Easy avocado curry with lentils

Afternoon snack: fresh vegetable greens, 1/4-caries

Denner: BANK granular and nos uinoina talked about dressing uikkum Cuminn Dressing

DESIGN: 1/2 cups from the collection
Sundays

The most important thing: VANILLA can pudding with 1 tablespoon of fresh beans

Lunh: Crisp red and green, looks like a little 1 tbsp sweet potatoes (or 1 small potato, packaged)

Afternoon snack: 1/4 cup hummingbird with fresh vegetables (horns, frogs, romantic leaves, balls, etc.)

FOOD : UNO INOALA BANK AND SALAD IN A FAST COMMUNITY PROJECT

STARTING UP PLANET BASE

Statistics show that more and more people are choosing herbal diets; People are aware of the benefits of a herbal diet. In the United States, over a third of consumers actively consume more plant products.

Celebrities like F1 champion Lewis Hamilton Will I Am, award-winning Hollywood director Ava DuVernay, screenwriter Alicia Silverstone, actor and musician Moby also supported the cause of the herbal diet.

Why Use A Vegetable Diet?

According to research and various studies, the herbal diet is known to prevent and reverse type II diabetes and advanced cardiovascular disease.

Studies have also shown that people on a plant-based diet can lose weight more easily, reduce the risk of sudden death, and reduce the risk of heart disease.

Doctors, nutritionists and health care professionals have combined the continued use of herbal diets to treat and prevent high (and bad) cholesterol, hypertension and the risk of certain types of cancer.

Academy of Nutrition and Dietetics found that in Las Vegas, a properly designed YEL this m ± ka, Spirit LNE vegetarian diet ñ ska ska and rock (including has the desired food, alcohol Kiro, vegetables), with a healthy diet, it is desirable nutritionally dense and the best for all to people regardless of age or regardless of age , regardless , such as childhood, adolescence, adulthood, pregnancy and old age, athletes can also choose this diet.

I am sure that the benefits will be affected. I mentioned it and I'm happy to get to the train; Despite the size of these points, you should realize that the transition is a bit difficult. Some people wanted to go but couldn't follow.

This means that your initial energy in the beginning must be strong enough to support you as you live this lifestyle. It means a lot of planning, willpower and commitment.

I had to tell my clients to move gradually. If you've been drinking soda and popcorn every day for the past 10 years, it may be almost impossible not to do so for a week.

Here are some simple strategies that have helped me and my customers a smooth transition HCl of herbal ä aqueous solution of the diet.

Start with small steps

Switching to a plant-based diet is no different than learning to walk on one foot for months on end. It is best to start with normally eaten vegetarian meals. It can be a burrito with beans and rice, oatmeal, three fried peppers, spring spaghetti, fried vegetables or lentils.

This way you can start gradually and develop these foods. It's a better way to choose this diet because only human nature is dedicated to our love. It is better to build slowly as it will relieve you of the pressure you initially know.

Decreased consumption of processed foods and meat.

Instead of cutting meat and processed foods, you can also reduce the consumption of animals and processed foods. Change the dimensions 80:20, 70:30, 60:40, 50:50, 45:55, 40:60, 30:70, 20:80, 10:90 to get a 100% vegetarian diet. The first set of numbers refers to processed foods, meat and animal products, and the second series refers to food of plant origin.

By doing this this way, you are giving your mind and body time to adjust to this diet. You can start by adding a few tablespoons of salad to your meal, then replace the meat with vegetable substitutes such as Portobello or dried Bulgarian mushrooms.

Start with a healthy herb for breakfast

After starting the first two steps, you can move on to the third step, which is a daily breakfast of vegetables. Make this your first meal of the day so that your body gradually warms up. After balance, go for lunch and then customize your snacks and dinners

Check your protein intake

While our bodies need about one gram of protein per kilogram of body weight, many people consume the desired amount of it daily.

The fact that the body needs protein is not a cause for excessive consumption as it can also be harmful to the body. All you have to do is find food that can provide you with the nine important amino acids your body really needs.

The good thing is that foods from healthy plants contain proteins and amino acids in different ratios. Once you've consumed the right amount of calories your body needs, it's easy to focus on whole foods. It also means that protein deficiency is severe.

You know what you're spending

You need to know what you are doing and how to make perfect and healthy meals for you. There are many plant products on the market, such as cheese and fakes, but they are very sophisticated. It can be very harmful to the body because it is highly saturated with saturated fats, amino acids, flour, salts, refined oils and sugars.

Therefore, it is best to know what you are buying and read the label before buying. Explore and select organic and whole products. Try ä read the nutrition and breeding s mit s sy o t. L ö will find s variety of ways to prepare various dishes.

If you can hire a vegetable nutritionist, help her plan and choose the best food for her. I had the opportunity to do it for people, which made it easier for my clients to switch. This lifestyle can be difficult, but with the help of a nutritionist, it is easy.

Healthy food will never stop

There are many healthy products that you can easily find by visiting the supermarkets and shops. This allows easier integration of plant products and lifestyle changes. There is milk without dairy products, tofu, potatoes and tempeh.

Whatever the price, you can still afford to go to the side aisles of vegetarian and fresh produce the next time you visit the supermarket. There is never a shortage of a healthy and nutritious diet; Keep some in your bag, drawers, workplace, refrigerator and worktop.

Be creative with what you eat

Start eating and learn how it works creatively. You can learn recipes and try something new for yourself; The more you try, the better you are. Discover new ways to prepare salads, soups, and daily use so you don't miss the time to serve the same every day.

Take snacks whenever you want (I'll show you how to make them in the following chapters). Take the time to learn recipes from different blogs and restaurants.

Find a group

Social media is easy to reach for just about anyone or anything. Find groups to help you learn and acquire new skills. They can encourage you when you need it and teach you what to do when your desires begin; You can also ask questions.

Usually you should be seen as a young child studying. This way you will not force yourself to learn. Find the one that suits you and stay with him.

ESTABLISHING BUILDING SERVICES The 50 most important food principles

We talked at length about what to eat, time to work. Now you need to know how to do what is really good for you. That is the only way to be 100% sure what you are eating.

I will teach you how to cook all vegetarian foods and what to do with vegetables, fruits, legumes, tubers, grains and other whole foods. I'll give you recipes for all kinds of foods around the world.

It doesn't matter if you are a beginner or a chef; I'm sure you will learn something new or something that can be improved. At some point I'm sure that you do wonders for your kitchen.

cash receipts

We use the information in the recipes and have fun. In the following chapters, I will give you over 100 recipes to help you find the flavors of vegetarian food, and I hope you love this lifestyle.

These recipes are free of cholesterol, low in saturated fats, balanced sodium and potassium, healthy heart and rich in antioxidants. While they all have immunostimulatory and anti-inflammatory properties, I will mention some turbo-charged recipes in this area due to some special ingredients that indicate which recipes are particularly suitable for children, without nuts, gluten and without quick preparation (15 minutes or less).

In addition to meal plans, there are many meals and delicious and nutritious desserts so you can enjoy healthy meals over long distances.

Max Power Shake

Produces 3-4 cups.

Preparation time: 5 minutes

Quick preparation without gluten pleasing to children Anti-inflammatory immunity enhancer

It's a great breakfast base to start the day with optional supplements to maximize nutrient density.

Shoots and fires can be difficult, so it is best to pull the leaves from the stem and work only with the leaves. Vegetables and carrots work best if you have an efficient blender such as Blendtec or Vitamix.

If you have a normal mixer, skip the fresh vegetables and use the green powder as a vegetable brand for brittle injections of nutrients.

- **1 banana**
- **¼ cup of oatmeal and 1 tablespoon of powdered protein**
- **1 tablespoon linseed or Chia seeds**
- **1 cup of raspberries or other berries**
- **1 cup chopped mango (frozen or fresh)**

- ½ cup raw milk (optional)
- 1 cup of water
  BONUS LEADERS (optional)
- 2 tablespoons fresh parsley or chopped basil
- 1 cup chopped fresh cabbage, spinach, cottage cheese or other vegetation
- 1 peeled carrot
- 1 tablespoon grated fresh ginger

1 Slide everything into a blender and add more water (or other milk) as needed

2 Add some, all, or all of the additional enhancements needed to mix the mix

Go ahead: buy more bananas to peel and put them in the freezer as an adult. Frozen bananas ensure maximum smoothness of the cocktail.

Chai Chia Shake

Prepare 3 desired cups

Preparation time: 5 minutes

Gluten Free PREPARATION FOR NEW INFLAMMATION

Chai spices can help digestion, improve glycemic control and increase metabolism. Chia seeds are a fantastic source of omega-3 fatty acids, calcium, phosphorus and manganese. Prepare these delicious cocktails to enjoy your trip as an alternative to the highly nutritious Lai Chai.

- **1 banana**
- **½ cup of coconut milk**
- **1 cup of water**
- **1 cup alfalfa sprouts (optional)**
- **1 to 2 soft, boneless Medjool dates**
- **1 tablespoon Chia seeds or ground flax or hemp**
- **¼ teaspoon ground cinnamon**
- **A pinch of ground cardamom**

- **1 tablespoon fresh grated ginger or 1/4 teaspoon ground ginger**

Clean everything in the blender evenly by adding more water (or coconut milk) as needed.

You know, though the dates are very sweet, they don't cause hyperglycemia. They have excellent additional HCl m HCl of sweets and add HCl m HCl of obtaining fibers and potassium.

TROPIKAL-breeze

Produces 3-4 cups.

Preparation time: 5 minutes

Quick preparation

Gluten free. Child-friendly. Anti-inflammatory immunity enhancer

Pineapple is a natural metabolic activator and contains an enzyme that helps digestion and reduce the bitterness of cabbage. If you 've never tried vegetables in a cocktail, try them first. You can turn the cabbage into a spinach if you want to start with a sweeter taste. We also use avocados to get sour cream instead of yellow banana. Today's decision is a low-carb carbohydrate option, see the yellow stew from other cocktails. Add a teaspoon of matcha green tea powder as needed to increase the dose.

- **1 cup chopped pineapple (frozen or fresh)**
- **1 cup chopped mango (frozen or fresh)**
- **½ up to 1 cup chopped cabbage**
- **½ avocado**
- **½ cup of coconut milk**

- **1 cup water or coconut water**
- **1 teaspoon matcha green tea powder (optional)**

Clean everything in the blender evenly by adding more water (or coconut milk) as needed.

Did you know that Matcha Green Tea Powder contains catechins that minimize inflammation and maximize fat burning potential?

irrigation station

Produces 3-4 cups.

Preparation time: 5 minutes

Fast confirmation

FRIENDS TO FRIEND FREE IRON

If you have a headache in the morning, it is a shock to you. Headaches are often a sign of dehydration, so increase the amount of water and electrolytes with this powerful and delicious shake. It is also ideal after training or competition to supplement and refresh.

- **1 banana**
- **1 peeled and chopped orange or 1 cup orange juice**
- **1 cup strawberries (frozen or fresh)**
- **1 cup chopped cucumber**
- **½ cups coconut water**
- **1 cup of water**
- **½ cup of ice**

BONUS LEADERS (optional)

- **1 cup chopped spinach**
- **¼ cup fresh mint, chopped**

1 Place everything in a blender evenly, adding water if necessary

2 Add bonus updates as needed. Mash confused

Advantage: Pour a cocktail into an insulated travel cup or thermos to keep cool while traveling

Mango madness

Produces 3-4 cups.

Preparation time: 5 minutes

Fast confirmation

FRIENDS TO FRIEND FREE IRON

Charge your immune system, which is rich in vitamin C. Cocktail is also rich in beta-carotene for sharp eyes and clean skin. If you don't have a strong blender or don't want a carrot in a cocktail, you can ignore it.

- 1 banana
- 1 cup chopped mango **(frozen or fresh)**
- 1 cup chopped peach **(frozen or fresh)**
- 1 cup of strawberries
- 1 carrot, peeled and **chopped (optional)**
- 1 cup of water

Rub everything in the mixer evenly, adding more water as needed

Alternatives: If you can't find frozen peaches and fresh peaches, this is not the

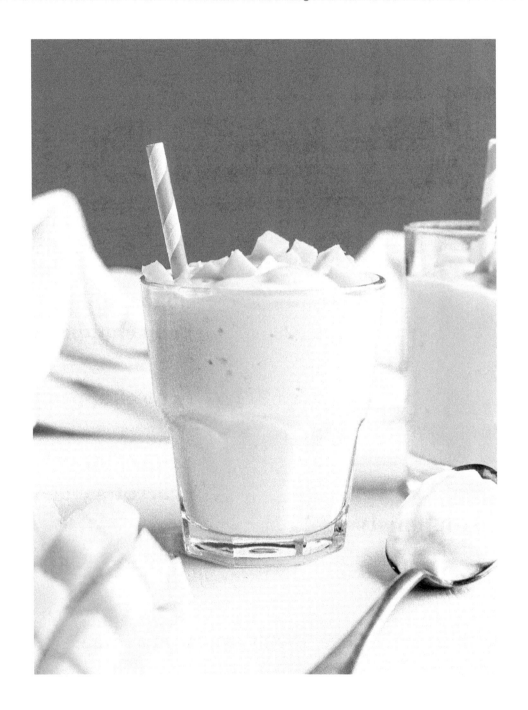

Milk Cocktail milk PB

Produces 3-4 cups.

Preparation time: 5 minutes

Quick preparation for children

This cocktail is so delicious that you may not think it healthy, but it is 100% good. It contains all the nutrients for a good start to the day, keeps it at dinner, and is the perfect counterbalance to Monday morning sadness.

- **1 banana**
- **¼ cup of oatmeal and 1 tablespoon of powdered protein**
- **1 tablespoon linseed or Chia seeds**
- **1 tablespoon bitter cocoa powder**
- **1 tablespoon peanut butter or almond butter or sunflower seeds**
- **1 tablespoon maple syrup (optional)**
- **1 cup alfalfa or chopped spinach (optional)**
- **½ cup raw milk (optional)**

- **1 cup of water**

BONUS LEADERS (optional)

1 teaspoon maca powder

1 teaspoon cocoa beans

1 Slide everything into a blender and add more water (or other milk) as needed

2 Add bonus updates as needed. Mash confused

Did you know that cocoa flavonols help protect the vascular mucosa , and postmenopausal women seem to have the greatest cardiac benefit of cocoa use?

Pink panther smoothie

Prepare 3 desired cups

Preparation time: 5 minutes

Fast confirmation without resistance to preparation to prevent you from driving fast

Cocktail is soft as silk, with little dynamics. Berries are a rich source of vitamin C and contain many unique nutrients that provide protection, antioxidants, anti-inflammatory and liver and prevent cancer (especially breast, colon, lung and prostate) and urinary tract infections.

- **1 cup of strawberries**
- **1 cup chopped melon** **(all types)**
- **1 cup of blueberries** **or raspberries**
- **1 tablespoon Chia seeds**
- **½ cups of coconut milk or other milk work**
- **1 cup of water**

BONUS LEADERS (optional)
1 teaspoon of goji-berry
2 tablespoons chopped fresh mint

instructions:

1 Slide everything in the blender until smooth, adding more water (or coconut milk) as needed

2 Add bonus updates as needed. Mash confused

Alternatives: If you don't have (or don't like) coconut, try sunflower seeds to increase zinc and selenium resistance

Banana-nut cocktail

Produces 2-3 cups.

Preparation time: 5 minutes

WITHOUT CHILDREN CHILDREN

It's like a banana bread in a glass. Prepare a quick breakfast or dessert. Almond butter is already creamy, but if you have a strong blender, it is also very tasty and contains 2 tablespoons of nuts instead of almond butter. Bowl with muesli or muesli and fresh fruit slices.

- **1 banana**
- **1 tablespoon almond butter or sunflower butter**
- **¼ teaspoon ground cinnamon**
- **A pinch of ground nutmeg**
- **1-2 tablespoons or maple syrup**
- **1 tablespoon flax, chia or hemp seeds**
- **½ cup raw milk (optional)**
- **1 cup of water**

Clean everything in the blender evenly by adding more water (or non-milk) as needed.

Options: You can make a pumpkin spice cocktail by adding 1 cup of cooked pumpkin and a pinch of allspice

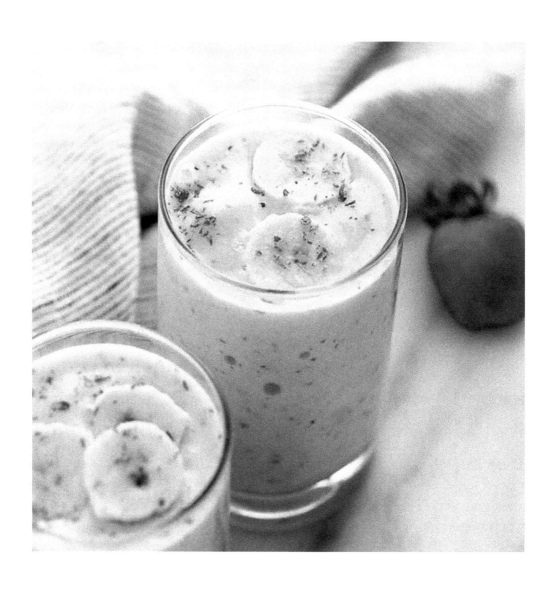

Oatmeal at night

Take one dose

Preparation time: 5 minutes / Cooking time: 5 minutes or overnight.

Gluten-free preparation without kids' friends

Oatmeal is known for its heart-protecting benefits. Beta-glucan fibers, which lower cholesterol by using only antioxidants, avantantamides, which can help cleanse blood vessel walls and lignans to protect against heart disease, are attractive packs. His basic porridge is practically a superhero.

AVENA GROUNDS FOR NIGHT

- ½ cup gluten-free oatmeal or quinoa
- 1 tablespoon ground flaxseeds, chia seeds or hemp seeds
- 1 tablespoon maple syrup or coconut sugar (optional)
- ¼ teaspoon ground cinnamon (optional)

OUT OF STOCK OPTIONS

- 1 chopped apple and 1 tablespoon nuts

- **2 tablespoons dried cranberries and 1 tablespoon pumpkin seeds**
- **1 chopped pear and 1 tbsp cashew**
- **1 cup chopped grapes and 1 tablespoon sunflower seeds**
- **1 chopped banana and 1 tablespoon peanut butter**
- **2 tablespoons raisins and 1 tablespoon hazelnuts**
- **1 cup blueberries and 1 tablespoon unsweetened coconut flakes**

1 Mix oat flakes, linseed, maple syrup and cinnamon (if used) in a bowl or take them (travel cup or short thermos works well)

2 Pour the oats in cold enough water to soak them and mix to combine. Soak for at least half an hour or overnight.

3 Add a region selection

Quick alternative in the morning: boil about ½ cup water and pour the oatmeal. Soak them for about 5 minutes before eating.

Did you know that cinnamon has been shown **to help** control blood sugar to improve insulin response and reduce

Breakfast cookies with oatmeal

Make 5 big cookies

Preparation time: 15 minutes / Cooking time: 12 minutes.

Quick preparation for children

Breakfast can be very healthy, even if you fry it in a cookie. Think of it as a bowl of healthy porridge, just for fun. Oatmeal, linseed, nuts and whole grains are good for cardiovascular health, so these cookies are the perfect start to the day. Make them gluten-free simply by using sorghum and oatmeal or quinoa instead of regular porridge.

- **1 tablespoon ground flax seeds**
- **2 tablespoons almond butter or sunflower butter**
- **2 tablespoons maple syrup**
- **1 banana puree**
- **1 teaspoon ground cinnamon**
- **¼ teaspoon nutmeg (optional)**
- **A pinch of sea salt**

- **½ cup of oatmeal**
- **¼ cup of dark chocolate raisins or shavings**
- 1 Preheat oven to 350 ° F. Place a large baking sheet on parchment paper

2 Mix the linen with enough water to cover it on a plate and set it aside

3 Mix the almond butter and maple syrup in a large bowl until creamy, then add the banana Add the linen and water mixture

4 Replace the cinnamon, nutmeg and salt in a separate medium bowl, then mix with the wet mixture

5 Add oatmeal and raisins and double

6 Make a ball with 3-4 tablespoons of pasta and lightly press to smooth the pan. Repeat from each other by separating o s steet 2 to 3 inches

7 Cook for 12 minutes or until golden

8 Store cookies in an airtight container in the refrigerator or freeze for later use

Keep on going: this number is for one person so you don't have many cakes to entice, but they are perfect for doubling your entire snack

Cupcakes in the sun

Make 6 muffins

Preparation time: 15 minutes / Cooking time: 30 minutes.

IMMEDIATELY Fast, Immediate INSTALLATION REQUIREMENT FOR CHILDREN

These cupcakes are the perfect starting point for the day, with plenty of flavors and nutrients. They have very little fat and added sugars based on healthy fruit candies. Add a few tablespoons of maple syrup to make it a little sweeter. Try combining a roll with a medium C or Hoi and ideas for a balanced breakfast.

- 1 teaspoon coconut oil to dispense muffins (optional)
- 2 tablespoons almond butter or sunflower butter
- ¼ cup of raw milk
- 1 peeled orange
- 1 carrot, cut into large pieces
- 2 tablespoons chopped dried apricots or other dried fruits
- 3 tablespoons molasses
- 2 tablespoons ground flax seeds

- vinegar
- vanilla extract
- cinnamon
- powder (optional)
- (optional)
- pepper (optional)
- whole jyvi s
- powder
- soda

1 teaspoon apple wine

1 teaspoon of pure

½ teaspoon ground

½ teaspoon of ginger

¼ teaspoon nutmeg

¼ teaspoon Jamaican

¾ cup of oatmeal or

1 teaspoon baking

½ teaspoon baking

ROLLERSIMET (OPTIONAL)

-
- or other dried fruits
- sunflower seeds

½ cup of oatmeal
2 tablespoons raisins

2 tablespoons

1 Preheat oven to 350 ° F. Prepare a 6-cup muffin bowl by rubbing the inside of the cups with coconut oil or using silicon cups or paper cups.

2 Clean peanut butter, milk, orange, carrot, apricots, molasses, linseed, vinegar, vanilla, cinnamon, ginger, nutmeg and spice in a cooker or blender.

3 Flour the oats in a clean coffee grinder until smooth (or use whole wheat flour). Combine the oatmeal in a large bowl with baking powder and baking soda.

4 Mix the wet ingredients with the dry ingredients until combined. Assemble accessories (if you use them)

5 Bake about ¼ cup of pasta on each loaf and bake for 30 minutes until the inside rod is clean. The orange forms a very moist base, which allows the rollers to last more than 30 minutes depending on the weight of the muffin.

Storage: Store muffins in the refrigerator or freezer as they are extremely moist. If you plan to keep them frozen, you can easily double the batch with a full dozen

Crisp apple and compote muffins

He makes 12 cups

Preparation time: 15 minutes / Cooking time: 15-20 minutes.

Quick preparation for children

They are customized from my childhood favorite sandwiches so that they are full of vegetables and low in fat and sugar. Coconut sugar is a great choice for a sweetener with a low glycemic index, but if you can't find it, choose raw brown sugar such as succinate, date sugar or other unrefined powdered sugar. Do not use brown sugar that is just refined white sugar by adding molasses, nutmeg, demerara or turbinate that has only been partially refined, so it would be nice.

- **1 teaspoon coconut oil to dispense muffins (optional)**
- **2 tablespoons peanut butter or seed butter**
- **1½ cups unsweetened apple mousse**
- **⅓ cup of coconut sugar**
- **½ cup raw milk**
- **2 tablespoons ground flax seeds**
- **1 teaspoon apple wine vinegar**

- 1 teaspoon of pure vanilla extract
- 2 cups whole grain flour
- 1 teaspoon baking soda
- ½ teaspoon baking powder
- 1 teaspoon round cinnamon
- A pinch of sea salt
- ½ cup chopped nuts
- Ingredients (optional)
- ¼ cup walnuts
- ¼ cups coconut sugar
- ½ teaspoon ground cinnamon

1 Preheat oven to 350 ° F. Prepare two 6-cup muffin trays by rubbing the inside of the cups with coconut oil or using silicon cups or paper cups.

2 In a large bowl, combine peanut butter, apple mousse, coconut sugar, milk, linseed, vinegar and vanilla until well blended or cleaned in a kettle or blender.

3 Strain another large bowl of flour, baking soda, baking powder, cinnamon, salt and chopped nuts

4 Mix the dry and wet ingredients until combined

5 Put about 1/4 cup of batter into each muffin and sprinkle with the topping you choose (if using). Bake for 15-20 minutes or until the inner stick is cleaned. Apple juice creates a very moist base so cupcakes can last longer depending on the weight of the cans.

Alternatives: If you want to do this without nuts, replace the nuts with sunflower seeds and use butter with sunflower seeds

French toast with bananas and raspberry syrup

This makes 8 Plasterk in bed a year

Preparation time: 10 minutes / Cooking time: 30 minutes.

QUICK PREPARATION FOR FREE KIDS 'FRIENDS

Making French toast with bananas instead of eggs gives it a natural sweetness and a new taste. You don't have to worry about baking it a little. Raspberry syrup Beauty lies in the fact that the sweetness of the berries means that only a small number of Œ of maple syrup, which reduces tool wit aj ± c ± number of SC added sugar.

French toast

- 1 banana
- 1 cup coconut milk
- 1 teaspoon of pure vanilla extract
- 1/4 teaspoon ground nutmeg
- ½ teaspoon ground cinnamon
- 1 ½ teaspoon plum powder or flour
- A pinch of sea salt
- 8 slices of whole wheat bread

RASPBERRY-SYRUPille

1 cup fresh or frozen raspberries or other berries

2 tablespoons water or pure fruit juice

1 or 2 tablespoons maple syrup or coconut sugar (optional)

FRENCH BREAD PRODUCTION

1 Preheat oven to 350 ° F.

2 Grate or grate banana in a shallow bowl, stir in coconut milk, vanilla, nutmeg, cinnamon, carrot and salt.

3 Dip the slices of bread into the banana mixture and then place them in a 13x9 inch baking mold. They should cover the bottom of the disc and may overlap slightly, but should not overlap. Pour bread with the remaining banana and place in the oven. Cook for about 30 minutes or until the work surface turns slightly brown.

4 Serve with raspberry syrup.

RASPBERRY-SYRUPIN TEE

1 Heat the raspberries in a small saucepan with water and maple syrup (if using) over medium heat

2 Cook over low heat, stirring and crushing the berries occasionally for 15 to 20 minutes, until the liquid is reduced.

Residues: Raspberry Residue Syrup is the perfect addition to a simple oatmeal for

breakfast or a quick and delicious season of whole grain toast with natural peanut butter

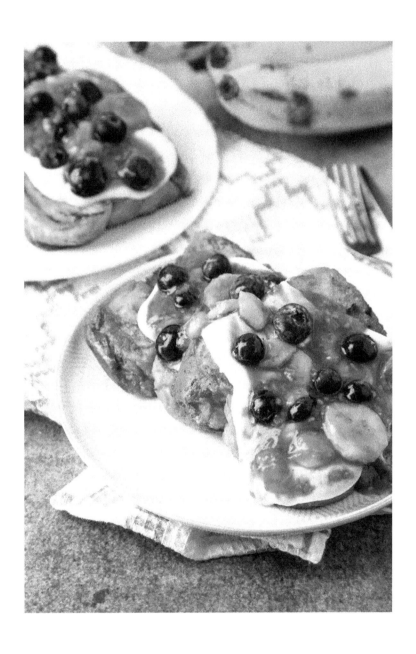

Toast with apple and cinnamon

Make 2 slices

Preparation time: 5 minutes / Cooking time: 10-20 minutes.

QUICK PREPARATION FOR FREE KIDS 'FRIENDS

This is a very simple decadent brunch. Apples help regulate blood glucose levels, reduce fat and cholesterol, and maintain the balance of intestinal flora. Apples contain a phytoremediation called quercetin, which has anti-inflammatory and antihistamine properties and is much more concentrated on the skin than on meat. In fact, apples contain many nutrients that focus on the skin, so you should eat them.

- **coconut oil**
- **cinnamon**
- **syrup or coconut sugar**
- **chopped**
- **wheat bread**

- **1-2 teaspoons of**
- **½ teaspoon ground**
- **1 tablespoon maple**
- **1 apple, heartless and**
- **2 slices of whole**

1 In a large bowl, combine coconut oil, cinnamon and maple syrup. Add apple slices and mix hands to cover

2 To bake the toast, place the apple slices in a medium saucepan over medium heat and cook for about 5 minutes until slightly soft, then transfer to a plate. Bake bread in the same pan for 2-3 minutes on each side. Cover the toast with apples. Alternatively, you can make a toast. Rub each piece of bread with a handful of coconut oil mixture on both sides with your hand . Place them on a baking sheet, cover with apples covered and place in oven or toaster at 350 ° F for 15 to 20 minutes or until apples are soft.

Alternatives: For a more relaxed version, bake bread, spread with peanut butter, cover with apple slices and sprinkle with cinnamon and coconut sugar.

A bowl of muesli and blueberries

It's about 5 cups

Preparation time: 10 minutes

Quick preparation for children

Muesli is a great alternative to muesli; It is less fat and does not cook. Health stores to find a whole , and p o rr o ISI s flakes: Find the smallest m HCl r s ingredients eik days additional days tty s sugar. It's a really tasty and energetic breakfast on weekdays as an alternative to oatmeal or cocktails. Pid s fun to experiment with different p s nut ö it ä , seeds, fruits and spices, which they may contain.

Example

- **1 cup oatmeal**
- **1 cup spelled, quinoa or oats**
- **2 cups blown cereal**
- **¼ cup of sunflower seeds**
- **¼ cup mantel**
- **¼ cup raisins**
- **¼ cup of dried cranberries**
- **¼ cup chopped dried figs**

- ¼ cup of unsweetened grated coconut
- ¼ cup milk chocolate
- 1-3 teaspoons ground cinnamon

CUENCOlle

- ½ cup of unsweetened milk or apple foam
- ¾ cup cups
- ½ cup of berries

1 Place the muesli ingredients in a bowl or bag and shake.

2 Combine the ingredients of the muesli and the bowl on a drawing pan or plate.

Compensation: try Brazilians p s nut o it s , peanut s nut ö it ä , dried cranberries, dried cranberries, dried mangoes or mit ä any time, MIK s inspires you. Ginger and cardamom are great flavors if you want to fork with spices.

Cinema and chocolate breakfast bowl

Take 2 doses

Preparation time: 5 minutes / Cooking time: 30 minutes.

Fast without gluten without friends

You can eat perfectly healthy desserts for breakfast. Quinoa is a great addition to your morning protein boost, but you can use any cooked wheat from oatmeal to brown rice. Pudding is also great chocolate as a snack or dessert.

- **1 cup of quinoa**
- **1 teaspoon ground cinnamon**
- **1 cup milk without milk**
- **1 cup of water**
- **1 big banana**
- **2-3 tbsp bitter cocoa powder or locust beans**
- **1 or 2 tablespoons almond butter or other peanut butter or seed butter**
- **1 tablespoon powdered linseed or Chia seeds or hemp**
- **2 tbsp nuts**
- **¼ cup of raspberries**

1 Put quinoa, cinnamon, milk and water in a medium saucepan. Cook over high heat, then lower the temperature and simmer for 25-30 minutes.

2 When mixing the quinoa, mix or grate the banana in a medium bowl and add the cocoa powder, almond butter and linseed.

3 To serve, pour 1 cup of boiled quinoa in a bowl, cover with half the pudding, half the walnuts and raspberries

Prepare in advance: This is a great way to use quinoa scraps or plan ahead and prepare extra quinoa for dinner so you can prepare it from morning to Monday with a milkshake

Carrot and ginger soup

Prepare 3 to 4 large bowls

Preparation time: 10 minutes / Cooking time: 20 minutes.

Quick preparation without gluten

Carrot and ginger soup is easy and easy to prepare during the week, it is also nutritious and really tasty. Carrots still have good eyesight due to their high beta-carotene content, but carrots have also been shown to contain antioxidants and other nutrients to protect against cardiovascular disease, cancer and liver problems. . Additions of white beans (mentioned here Cannellini beans, which is white beans, but works with all kinds of white beans) makes the soup is full of wit, strong, creamy and rich in spirit white wit ego box wit each.

- **1 teaspoon of olive oil**
- **1 cup chopped onion**
- **1 tablespoon chopped fresh ginger**
- **4 large carrots, peeled or rubbed and chopped (about 2 cups)**
- **1 cup cannellini beans cooked or canned and washed or other delicate white Papua**
- **½ cup vegetable broth or water and add salt**
- **2 glasses of water**

- **¼ teaspoon of sea salt**

1 Heat olive oil in large saucepan, fry onion and ginger for 2-3 minutes. Add the carrots and cook until tender, about 3 minutes.

2 Add the beans, vegetable broth, water and salt and simmer for 20 minutes.

3 Transfer the soup to a blender or mass with a dipping mixer. Serve hot.

Residues : Store the **residue in** an airtight container in the refrigerator for one week or in the freezer for one or two months.

Coconut soup with watercress

Makes 4 bowls

Preparation time: 10 minutes / Cooking time: 20 minutes.

Fast confirmation without resistance to preparation to prevent you from driving fast

These mixed soups are the perfect way to collect many incognito vegetables. This soup is so delicious that no one complains about eating vegetables, and its cream SC is s wit sweet wit, and alcohol in coconut milk compensates for the bitterness of watercress. To prepare ® for this recipe raw, use 2-3 regular meals, do not fry the onion and stir in the soup when it is cold.

- **1 teaspoon coconut oil**
- **1 chopped onion**
- **2 cups fresh or frozen peas**
- **4 cups water or vegetable broth**
- **1 cup fresh cress, chopped**
- **1 tablespoon chopped fresh mint**
- **A pinch of sea salt**
- **A pinch of freshly ground black pepper**

- **¾ cups of coconut milk**

1 Melt the coconut oil in a large saucepan over medium heat. Add the onions and cook until tender, about 5 minutes, add peas and water.

2 Bring to a boil, then lower the heat and add the cress, mint, salt and pepper. Cover and simmer for 5 minutes.

3 Add the coconut milk and stir until smooth in a blender or hand blender.

Alternatives: Try this soup made with fresh and leafy vegetables, spinach and cabbage, arugula and swiss lacquer

Beetroot and sweet potato soup

There are 6 bowls

Preparation time: 10 minutes / Cooking time: 30 minutes.

Quick preparation without gluten pleasing to children Anti-inflammatory immunity enhancer

This potato and beetroot recipe is easy to prepare and has an unusual taste. The combination of beets and sweet potatoes gives a rich taste and a thick, creamy texture. The soup has a pleasant beetroot color and is very hot on a cold afternoon.

- **5 cups unsalted water or vegetable broth (if salted, leave sea salt underneath)**
- **1-2 teaspoons olive oil or vegetable broth**
- **1 cup chopped onion**
- **3 ground garlic cloves**
- **1 tablespoon thyme, fresh or dried**
- **1-2 teaspoons of pepper**
- **2 cups peeled and chopped beets**
- **2 cups peeled and chopped sweet potatoes**
- **2 cups parsnip, peeled and chopped**

- ½ teaspoon of sea salt
- 1 cup chopped fresh mint
- ½ avocado or 2 tablespoons peanut butter or seed butter (optional)
- 2 tablespoons balsamic vinegar (optional)
- 2 tablespoons pumpkin seeds

1 Boil water in a large saucepan.

2 Heat another olive oil in a large saucepan and fry onion and garlic until tender, about 5 minutes.

3 Add thyme, peppers, beets, sweet potatoes and parsnips, and boiling water and salt. Cover and simmer for about 30 minutes until vegetables are soft.

4 Book a little mint for decoration and add the rest of the avocado (if used). Stir until well blended.

5 Transfer the soup to the blender or add the balsamic vinegar (if used) to the puree.

6 offer the pumpkin seeds and fresh mint and, where appropriate, with one side of the avocado pieces.

Residues: This soup is ideal for preparing and storing large quantities in single-dose containers in a freezer for a quick meal within a week

Miso noodle soup

Makes 4 bowls

Preparation time: 10 minutes / Cooking time: 15 minutes.

Gluten Free PREPARATION FOR NEW INFLAMMATION

Miso soup is Japanese and is traditionally served in the simplest way possible: broth, miso, seaweed, tofu cubes and shallots. Japanese miso soups in Japan also contain sardines and tuna in broth, but we consider them herbs. We will also connect. an approach that combines the concept of North American chicken soup with Japanese ingredients by purifying azuki beans and earthy Soba noodles (Soba is usually in small packs and 7 ounces is about two packs in a typical package).

- **7 ounces of soba pasta (use 100% gluten-free buckwheat)**
- **4 glasses of water**
- **4 tablespoons miso**
- **1 cup of azuki beans (cooked or canned), drained and rinsed**
- **2 tablespoons fresh coriander or chopped basil**
- **2 shallots, finely chopped**

1 Boil a large pot of water and occasionally add Soba Stir noodles; Cooking takes about 5 minutes.

In the meantime, prepare the rest of the soup by heating the water in a separate pot just below the boiling temperature and then remove from the heat. Add miso in water until it dissolves.

3 After cooking, rinse the pasta and rinse with hot water.

4 Add cooked noodles, azuki beans, coriander and chives to the miso broth and serve.

Technically: miso is a fermentation product and good brands have live microbial cultures such as yogurt, so it should be added to the broth when it's hot, not hot. Adding mise to boiling water changes the taste

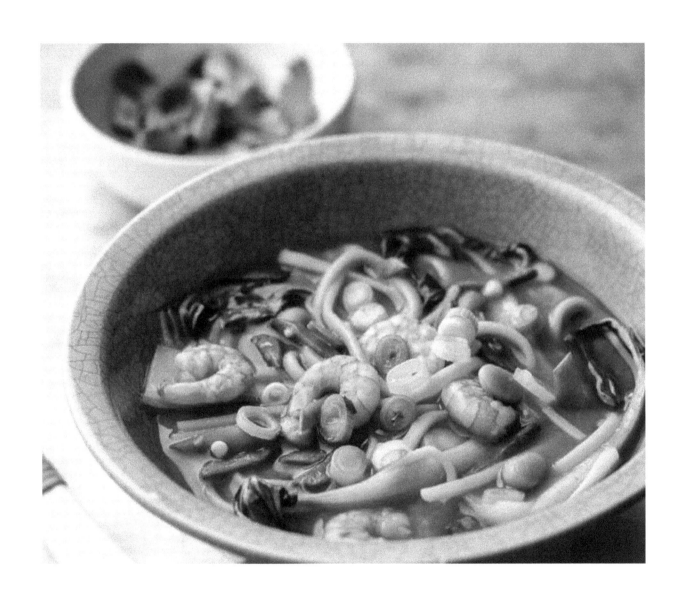

Puree pumpkin with large f folded nuts

Makes 4 bowls

Preparation time: 15 minutes / Cooking time: 30 minutes.

Quick confirmation without gluten without veterinary preparation

It is the perfect soup for warming and satisfying, helping the body to cleanse. It is very tasty and very rich, but gives the impression of concentrating books. It's the perfect spirit book for spiritual meals after the holidays when we ate last night and wanted too much.

- **1 small pumpkin pie, peeled, sown and chopped (about 6 cups)**
- **1 teaspoon of olive oil**
- **¼ teaspoon of sea salt**
- **1 chopped onion**
- **4 cups water or vegetable broth**
- **2-3 teaspoons of ground sage**
- **2-3 tablespoons of yeast**
- **1 cup milk or 1 tablespoon peanut butter or seed butter and 1 cup water or broth**

- **¼ cup of roasted nuts**

Fresh ground black pepper

1) Place the large saucepan at medium temperature and fry the pumpkin in oil, seasoning with salt for a light texture, about 10 minutes. Add the onion to the pan and cook until soft, about 5 minutes.

2 Add water and cook. Then lower the temperature to low heat, cover and cook for 15-20 minutes until the pumpkin softens after biting the fork

3 Add sage, nutritious yeast and non-milk. Then grate the soup with a dipping mixer or a regular blender

4 Garnish with roasted nuts and pepper.

Substitution: A winter pumpkin or sweet potato would be a great alternative to pumpkin in terms of structure, taste and nutrients.

Grilled peppers and pumpkin soup

There are 6 bowls

Preparation time: 10 minutes / Cooking time: 40-50 minutes.

Quick preparation without gluten pleasing to children Anti-inflammatory immunity enhancer

Grilled vegetables attract sugars and give this soup its full flavor. Vegetable cooking is the beauty of it, the cooking , placing them in the oven and other tasks making takes time . It's great that you have such a thick, creamy and tasty non-dairy soup.

- 1 small pumpkin
- 1 tablespoon olive oil
- 1 teaspoon sea salt
- 2 red peppers
- 1 yellow onion
- 1 head of garlic
- 2 cups water or vegetable broth
- 1 peel and lime juice
- 1-2 tablespoons of Tahini
- A touch of cayenne pepper
- ½ teaspoon of coriander powder

- **½ teaspoon ground cumin**
- **Roasted Pumpkin Seeds (Optional)**

1 Preheat oven to 350 ° F.

2 Prepare a fried pumpkin, cut it in half lengthwise, remove the seeds and make a fork with several holes in the flesh, preserving the seeds if necessary. Rub a small amount of oil on the flesh and skin, then rub in a little sea salt and place on a large pan. Put in the oven, cook the rest of the vegetables.

3 Prepare the peppers in exactly the same way except they do not have to be cut. Cut the onion in half and rub the oil on the bare sides. Cut the garlic tip and rub the oil on the bare meat.

4 After developing the pumpkin for 20 minutes, add the peppers, onions and garlic and cook for another 20 minutes. You can also toast pumpkin seeds by placing them on a separate plate in the oven   Spread 10-15 minutes before cooking vegetables. Watch them carefully.

5 After cooking, remove vegetables and allow to cool before using. The pumpkin is very sweet after the fork piercing.

Remove the meat from the pumpkin skin in a large saucepan (if you have an immersion blender) or in a blender. Finely chop the pepper, remove the onion peel and onion, squeeze the garlic clove on your head, all in a saucepan or blender, add water, lemon zest, juice and Tahini. Add soup, adding water to the desired consistency if needed.

7 Season with salt, pepper, coriander and cumin. Serve fried with pumpkin seeds (if used).

Did you know that winter day squash is high in vitamin A, which is good for eye health and skin repair and maintenance? It also strengthens the immune system. According to Chinese medicine, the winter base improves the circulation of Qi energy, which is its vitality

Tomato soup and chick peas on weekdays

Take 2 doses

Preparation time: 10 minutes / Cooking time: 20 minutes.

WARNING GLUTINITON-FREE RESISTANT Fast wheat production

This soup is quick and easy to prepare, as well as a very tasty, rich and wonderful flavor. It's perfect for a quick dinner during the week and enough for your next day's lunch. If you cook at least two, the recipe will double or triple.

- **1-2 teaspoons olive oil or vegetable broth**
- **½ cup chopped onion**
- **3 ground garlic cloves**
- **1 cup chopped mushrooms**
- **⅛ - ¼ teaspoon of sea salt divided**
- **1 tablespoon dried basil**
- **½ tablespoon dried oregano**
- **1 or 2 tablespoons of balsamic vinegar or red wine**
- **A can of dried tomatoes**

- **1 jar (14 ounces) of chickpeas, drained and rinsed, or 1 cup of cooked fats**
- **2 glasses of water**
- **1 or 2 cups chopped cabbage**

1 Heat a large olive oil in a large saucepan and fry onion, garlic and mushrooms with a pinch of salt until soft for 7 to 8 minutes.

2 Add the basil and oregano and stir to mix. Then add the vinegar to melt the pan with a wooden spoon to scrape all the salted and golden pieces from the bottom.

3 Add the tomatoes and chickpeas. Stir, combine, add enough water to obtain the desired consistency.

4 Add the cabbage and the remaining salt. Cover and simmer for 5-15 minutes until cabbage is as soft as you want.

Sauce: Delicious covered with a spoon of roasted nuts and a touch of nutritious yeast or sprinkled cheese

Abundant chili

Makes 4 bowls

Preparation time: 10 minutes / Cooking time: 10-20 minutes.

Fast Profit Fast Profit

Beans are an excellent source of protein, containing fiber, folic acid, iron and manganese, which lower cholesterol and stabilize blood glucose without saturated fat and ground beef cholesterol. The combination of iron-rich beans tomatoes rich in vitamin C and coriander means that .Pochod ¼ farther behind desired for the following for the desired iron, kt yellow re-correlates wi ± maximizes ± energy ê ± .

- **1 chopped onion**
- **2-3 ground garlic cloves**
- **1 teaspoon olive oil or 1 or 2 tablespoons water, vegetable fat or red wine**
- **1 can of tomato (28 ounces)**
- **¼ cup tomato paste or crushed tomato**
- **1 jar (14 ounces) of beans, rinsed and dried or 1 ½ cup for baking**
- **2-3 teaspoons chili powder**
- **¼ teaspoon of sea salt**

- **¼ cup of fresh cilantro or parsley leaves**

1 Fry the onions and garlic in the oil in a large saucepan for about 5 minutes. After softening, add the tomatoes, tomato paste, beans and chili powder. Season with salt.

2 Bake for at least 10 minutes or as long as you like. The flavors improve, the more they cook at low heat and even better, like the residue.

3 Garnish with coriander and serve.

Options: other papuilla have similar nutrients, so you can change them s you want. Try black beans, adzuki or black beans. Season with hot sauce if desired.

Indian red lentil soup

Makes 4 bowls

Preparation time: 5 minutes / Cooking time: 50 minutes.

Fast confirmation without resistance to preparation to prevent you from driving fast

It is a rich and hearty soup, which is a bold and warm taste of fresh ginger and Indian spices, such as coriander, cumin and turmeric. Sweet potatoes includes s lt s v s t rich in vitamin A, add HCl v s t delicate days of sweetness to stop the spices and vihannesjuurina to grinding and makes the s m HCl 's mind.

- **1 cup red lentils ä**
- **2 glasses of water**
- **1 teaspoon curry powder and 1 tablespoon split or 5 coriander seeds (optional)**
- **1 teaspoon coconut oil or 1 tablespoon water or vegetable fat**
- **1 red onion into cubes**
- **1 tablespoon chopped fresh ginger**
- **2 cups sweet potatoes, peeled and diced**
- **1 cup zucchini slices**

- **Fresh ground black pepper**
- **sea salt**
- **3-4 cups of vegetable broth or water**
- **1 or 2 teaspoons of toasted sesame oil**
- **1 bunch of chopped spinach**
- **Sesame Toast**

1 Put the lentils in a large saucepan with 2 glasses of water and 1 teaspoon of curry powder. Boil the lenses, then reduce the heat and simmer for 10 minutes until the lenses are soft.

2 Meanwhile, heat a large saucepan over medium heat, add the coconut oil and fry the onions and ginger until tender, about 5 minutes. Add the sweet potatoes and leave them on fire for about 10 minutes to soften slightly, then add the zucchini and cook until light, about 5 minutes. Add the remaining spoonful of curry powder, pepper and salt and stir in the vegetables to cover.

3 Add the vegetable broth, bring to a boil, then simmer cook and cover. Cook the vegetables slowly for 20 to 30 minutes or until the sweet potatoes soften.

4 Add the cooked lentils to the soup. Add another pinch of salt, toasted sesame oil and spinach. Stir, allowing spinach to dry before removing pan from heat.

5 Serve with roasted sesame seeds.

<u>Did you know that</u> <u>sweet potatoes made from orange pulp are tasty and are often called sweet potatoes even though technically white and orange potatoes are technically sweet? True yams are tropical tubers and are not generally sold in North America.</u>

Curry lentil burger

Produces 12 hamburgers.

Preparation time: 40 minutes / Cooking time: 30-40 minutes.

Gluten-free anti-inflammatory immune stimulator

When I started making vegetarian hamburgers, I tried to get a good texture that was good to keep but not too heavy. I tried many recipes before combining some aspects in my version, using carrots and many spices to lighten the lentils. These burgers are thick and rich, with tons of flavor and nutrition.

- **1 cup lenses**
- **2½ - 3 glasses of water s**
- **3 grated carrots**
- **1 small onion into cubes**
- **¾ cup whole grain flour (see gluten free options below)**
- **1 ½ or 2 teaspoons of curry powder**
- **½ teaspoon of sea salt**
- **A pinch of freshly ground black pepper**

1 Place the lentils in a medium bowl of water, cook and simmer for about 30 minutes.

2 When cooking lentils, place the carrots and onions in a large bowl. Mix with flour, curry, salt and pepper.

3 When the lentil is cooked, drain excess water and then add the vegetables to the bowl. Gently grate them with a grinder or large spoon and add more flour if you want the mixture to stick. The amount of flour depends on the amount of water absorbed by the lenses and the consistency of the flour, so use it roughly until the mixture adheres as the balls form. Remove 1/4 from the ministry and create 12 empanadas.

4You can bake or cook burgers. Paistaksesi warm a large pan over medium heat, add oil and cook hamburgers about 10 minutes at the first days isell s page. C HCl nn s CAP s r and cook s still days 5-7 minutes. Bake them, place them on a parchment lined plate and bake at 350 ° F for 30 to 40 minutes.

Alternatives: Use wholegrain flour, rice, oatmeal, buckwheat and even almond flour for gluten-free meal. The flour in this recipe is just an accident, so it can be any kind

Dijon hamburger maple

Produces 12 hamburgers.

Preparation time: 20 minutes / Cooking time: 30 minutes.

Reflective amplifier for children

Vegetarian burger fun is what you decide to spend. You can mix and match the burger to the sauce to your liking. They go well with marinade, avocado, cherry tomatoes and lettuce.

- 1 red pepper
- 1 can of washed and dried chick peas or 2 cooked cups
- 1 cup chopped almonds
- 2 teaspoons Dijon mustard
- 2 teaspoons maple syrup
- 1 garlic clove, pressed
- ½ lemon juice
- 1 teaspoon dried oregano
- ½ teaspoon dried sage
- 1 cup spinach
- 1-1½ cups of oatmeal

1 Preheat oven to 350 ° F. Place a large baking sheet on parchment paper.

2. Cut the pepper in half, removing the seeds and stem and then place the pan with the cut side of the furnace. Cook, preparing the rest of the ingredients.

3 Cook the chickpeas with almonds, mustard, maple syrup, garlic, lemon juice, oregano, sage and spinach. Press until everything is connected but clean. When the pepper softens slightly, about 10 minutes, add it to the oatmeal maker and press until sliced enough to create empanadas.

4 If you do not have a cooking appliance, mix the chickpeas with a meat grinder or fork and make sure everything else is chopped as finely as possible, and then mix.

5 Cut 1/4 cup portions and make 12 empanadas and place on a baking tray.

6 Place the burgers in the oven and cook until light brown for about 30 minutes.

Technique: It is important that you do not rub the ingredients because you want a hamburger texture, not a porridge. Use short pulses in the processor until the ingredients are chopped

Cajun Burger

Produces 5-6 hamburgers.

Preparation time: 25 minutes / Cooking time: 10-30 minutes.

ANTIPAL NUT GLUTE FREE

These burgers are made from grilled buckwheat (also known as porridge), which contains a routine flavonoid, contains plant lignans and is a good source of magnesium. All the heart-protecting nutrients in buckwheat can also help control your blood sugar. Combine this nutrition with incredible flavors. Turn them into a hamburger and get one of the best meals.

DRESS

- 1 tbsp Tahini
- 1 tablespoon apple wine vinegar
- 2 teaspoons Dijon mustard
- 1 or 2 tablespoons water
- 1 or 2 pressed garlic cloves
- 1 teaspoon dried basil
- 1 teaspoon dried thyme
- ½ teaspoon dried oregano

- ½ teaspoon dried sage
- ½ teaspoon smoked paprika
- ¼ teaspoon of cayenne pepper
- ¼ teaspoon of sea salt
- A pinch of freshly ground black pepper
- for Hamburg
- 2 glasses of water
- 1 cup manna (roasted buckwheat)
- A pinch of sea salt
- 2 grated carrots
- A handful of chopped fresh parsley
- 1 teaspoon olive oil (optional)

MAKE A SECURITY

1 In a medium bowl, combine Tahini, vinegar and mustard until very thick. Add 1 or 2 tablespoons of dilution water and mix again until smooth.

2 Add the rest of the ingredients. Reserve the flavors to mix.

IN HAMBURG

1 Pour water, buckwheat and sea salt into a medium saucepan. Simmer for 2-3 minutes, then simmer, cover and simmer for 15 minutes. The buckwheat is fully cooked when it is soft and there is no liquid in the bottom of the pan. Do not mix buckwheat during cooking.

2 When the buckwheat is cooked, transfer it to a large bowl. Combine grated carrots, fresh parsley and buckwheat sauce. Take a ¼ cup to serve and design hamburgers.

3 You can bake or cook burgers. Paistaksesi warm up a big pot over medium heat, add 1 teaspoon of olive oil and cook the burgers for about 5 minutes in the first days isell s page. C HCl nn s CAP s r and cook s still days 5 minutes. Keitt HCl skip to them, place them on a parchment lined baking-oven and bake at 350 ° F for about 30 minutes.

You know that buckwheat is not related to wheat. In fact, it is a grain and does not contain gluten. It also has a different nutritional profile than whole grains. Buckwheat is high in lysine amino acids, which helps to balance the plant's diet, as many vegetarian foods are high in other amino acids but low in lysine. Other lysine-rich foods include beans and pulses, quinoa and pistachios.

Grilled AHLT

He makes one sandwich

Preparation time: 5 minutes / Cooking time: 10 minutes.

Quick preparation without a child test

Give your BLT a healthy and delicious touch, replace bacon and avocado hummus. When grilling, the trade spinach was also a salad. If necessary, you can also use rubbed cabbage, rubbing it with your fingers until it dries and slightly moisten. It's the perfect place for a quick dinner with French.

- **¼ cup of classic hummus**
- **2 slices of whole wheat bread**
- **¼ avocado cutlet**
- **½ cup chopped salad**
- **½ chopped tomato**
- **A pinch of sea salt**
- **A pinch of freshly ground black pepper**
- **1 teaspoon olive oil, divided**

1 Spread some humus on each slice of bread. Then place the avocado, salad and tomato on a slice, sprinkle with salt and pepper and cover with another slice.

2 Heat a frying pan over medium heat and sprinkle headache with a spoon olive o Oil ä just before a cheese burger s The setting of the pan. Keit s 3 to 5 minutes, then take out sandwiches s plate, sprinkle half a teaspoon of olive o Oil LP , which is a j s ljell days in a saucepan, and rev s sandwich with the other half to boil 3 to 5 minutes. Close the vegetables with a spatula on the spa.

3 When done, remove pan and cut in half to serve.

Technique: You can also toast and fold it like a regular sandwich, or spread the bread on olive oil, fold the sandwich and put it on the toaster for 10-15 minutes at 350 ° F.

Loaded black bean pizza

Prepare 2 small pizzas

Preparation time: 10 minutes / Cooking time: 10-20 minutes.

FAST STRENGTHENING FRIENDS Friends' resistance to gluten free

This pizza is not only very tasty, but also full of delicious fresh vegetables. You can cook it or try it with ingredients to make it summer. Using bean sauce in pizza sauce will give you a dose of protein. There are many options for barking here. Go to the store with two hazelnuts or a complete package or create them yourself in Easy DIY Pizza Dough or Herbed Millet Pizza Dough, divided into two pizzas.

- **2 ready made pizza bases**
- **½ cup spicy black bean sauce**
- **1 tomato, thinly sliced**
- **A pinch of freshly ground black pepper**
- **1 grated carrot**
- **A pinch of sea salt**
- **1 red onion, finely chopped**
- **1 slice of avocado**

1 Preheat oven to 400 ° F

2 Place two skins on a large baking sheet. Spread half of the spicy black bean sauce on each pizza dough. Then add layers of tomato, if necessary with pepper and pepper.

3 Carefully sprinkle grated carrots with sea salt and sage. Spread the carrot on the tomato and then add the onion.

4 Put the pizzas in the oven for 10-20 minutes or until it responds.

5 Cover the cooked pizza with slices of avocado and another pepper.

Alternatives: Try making fresh zzz without cooking. Just load the pita or cook the skin before loading. You can use asparagus instead of red bonus points and taste if they are fresh alfalfa sprouts.

Mediterranean hummus pizza

Prepare 2 small pizzas

Preparation time: 10 minutes / Cooking time: 20-30 minutes.

Quick preparation without gluten pleasing to children Anti-inflammatory immunity enhancer

This is one of his favorite dishes of the week at home, as everything is available to the public and is quickly prepared for a satisfying meal. Organize your past pizzas with vegetables: Create what you want. Pizza is tasty and tasty, but if you don't want to try sun-dried and sun-dried tomatoes. You can use two pizzas or a package with a full peel, or you can do it yourself with Easy DIY pizza or Herbed Millet pizza envelope, split into two pizzas.

- **½ finely chopped zucchini**
- **½ chopped red onion**
- **1 cup cherry tomatoes, divided into two parts**
- **2-4 tablespoons chopped and chopped black olives**
- **A pinch of sea salt Olive Oil Shower (Optional)**
- **2 ready made pizza bases**

- **½ cup of classic hummus or roasted pepper hummus**
- **2 - 4 tablespoons grated cheese**

1 Preheat oven to 400 ° F.

2 Put my cucumbers, onions, cherry tomatoes and olives in a large bowl, sprinkle with sea salt and mix gently. Sprinkle a little olive oil (if used) to preserve flavor and prevent drying in the oven.

3 Place two skins on a large baking sheet. Apply half of the blemishes to each skin and cover with a mixture of herbs and a touch of cheese flakes.

4 Put the pizza in the oven for 20-30 minutes or until the vegetables are soft.

Prep : Gently cook the vegetables briefly before placing them in the pizza and cook for a few minutes until warm. I can even use other fried vegetables

Chickpea curry and mango package

There are 3 changes

Preparation time: 15 minutes

Quick preparation without a child test

Sweet mango combined with curry and flavored with calcium rich tachy is perfect. Eat it for dinner; You can heat vegetables and chickpeas before packing them and then pack the leftovers for lunch. Be sure to bring towels as they are a little dirty.

- 3 tbsp Tahini
- 1 peel and lime juice
- 1 tablespoon of curry powder
- ¼ teaspoon of sea salt
- 3-4 tablespoons of water
- 1 jar (14 ounces) of rinsed and dried chick peas or 1 ½ cup for baking
- 1 cup cubes of mango
- 1 red pepper, inoculated and diced
- ½ cup fresh coriander, chopped
- 3 large whole tablets 1-2 cups grated green salad

1 In a medium bowl, combine the Tahini, peel and lime juice, curry and salt until creamy and thick. Add 3-4 tablespoons of water to slightly dilute it . Or you can handle everything in the blender. The taste should be strong and salty to taste for each salad.

2 Stir in chickpeas, mangoes, pepper and coriander in Tahini sauce.

3 Cover the salad in the middle of the package, cover with the chopped salad, then roll and season.

Alternatives: replace salad leaves with integrated packaging. Use a hard salad such as Boston salad, Bibb salad or butter salad, or place an ornament on the escaroles if it fits a bit bitter

Falafel package

Prepare 6 cakes, 1 bag

Preparation time: 30 minutes / Cooking time: 30-40 minutes.

NOT a child friendly NUTS immune stimulator

Falafel and hummus are probably the most popular coffee specialties in the world, so combine them. Fill the falafel with nutritious additives such as parsley and cook or fry instead of frying vegetables. This recipe is meant to be packaged, but since falafel takes time, the recipe contains six biscuits that are enough for six wraps. Just pack more for the whole group, or give you some advice on what to do with the remaining falafel.

Falafel RATAKAT

- **1 jar (14 ounces) of chickpeas, drained and rinsed, or 1 cup of cooked fats**
- **1 grated courgette**
- **2 chives, chopped**
- **¼ cup fresh parsley, chopped**
- **2 tablespoons black olives, crushed and chopped (optional)**
- **1 tablespoon tahini or almond butter, cashew nuts or sunflower seeds**
- **1 tablespoon lemon juice or apple wine vinegar**

- cumin
- (optional if fried) package
- or pita
- hummus
- vegetables
-
- in half
- cucumber
- avocado or guacamole
- or cooked tabule (optional)

½ teaspoon ground

¼ teaspoon pepper

¼ teaspoon of sea salt

1 teaspoon olive oil

1 integrated package

¼ cup of classic

½ cup of fresh

1 baked falafel cake

¼ cup cherry tomato

¼ cup cubes of

¼ cup chopped

¼ cup quinoa salad

MAKE A FAULT

1 Add chickpeas, zucchini, shallots, parsley and olives (if necessary) in a cooking machine until chopped. Just press, don't delete. Or

mix the chickpeas in a large bowl with a meat grinder and add the grated and chopped vegetables.

2 Combine the batter and lemon juice in a small bowl and add the cumin, pepper and salt. Pour the chickpeas into the mixture and mix well (or press the cooker) to combine. If necessary, try adding more salt. Use your hands to form a mixture of 6 spans.

3 You can bake or bake a cake. To bake, heat a large frying pan over medium heat, add 1 teaspoon olive oil and cook dough for about 10 minutes on first page. Turn over and cook for another 5-7 minutes. Bake them, place them on a parchment lined plate and bake at 350 ° F for 30 to 40 minutes.

package

1 Place the package on a plate and spread the hummus in the middle. Then lie on the green and crumble the falafel cake on top. Add the tomatoes, cucumbers, avocados and quinoa.

2 Turn both ends and wrap as tightly as possible. If you have a sandwich press, you can press the pack for about 5 minutes. It is best to travel in reusable containers or reusable plastic containers.

Storage: Keep the remaining empanadas in a closed container in the refrigerator for one week or in the freezer for up to two months. Take them hamburger, season with your favorite spices (vegetables and beans

Pad Thai bowl

Makes 2 bowls

Preparation time: 10 minutes / Cooking time: 10 minutes.

GLUTEN Quick Prep Immune Response

Thai rhizomes are usually made with egg-fish sauce, which makes it difficult for vegetarians to find a solution. But don't worry because you can create your own taste and saturate as many flavors as you like compared to the restaurant version. In addition, you can pack a lot of fresh and tasty vegetables to increase nutrient density. Instead of the usual peanuts on top , you can pour this type of peanut directly into the sauce and drink it.

- **7 ounces of brown rice noodles**
- **1 teaspoon olive oil or 1 tablespoon vegetable broth or water**
- **2 carrots, peeled or rubbed and chopped in Julienne**
- **1 cup chopped pepper or red cabbage**
- **1 paprika, chopped and chopped**

- 2 shallots, finely chopped
- 2-3 tablespoons fresh mint, chopped
- 1 cup bean sprouts
- ¼ cup peanut sauce
- ¼ cup chopped fresh coriander
- 2 tablespoons grilled peanuts, chopped
- Fresh lime wedges

1 Place the rice noodles in a large bowl or saucepan and cover with boiling water. Let it soften for about 10 minutes. Rinse, filter and cool.

Heat oil in medium saucepan and fry carrots, cabbage and pepper until tender, 7-8 minutes. Add the shallots, mint and beans and cook for a minute or two, then remove from heat.

3 Mix the pasta with the vegetables and mix with the nuts sauce.

4 Transfer to bowls and sprinkle with coriander and peanuts.

Serve a slice of lime to squeeze the dish and give it a taste.

Alternatives: Try a richer version of this bowl, bake rice noodles and peel, or turn zucchini or carrot into a long "spaghetti"

Bowl of coconut dragon

There is 1 bowl

Preparation time: 10 minutes / Cooking time: 20 minutes.

QUICK PREPARATION FREE INFLAMMATIC GLUTEN

This salty and creamy bowl is easy to make but tasty and nutritious. It does not contain oil, but the fat content of coconut makes months ± ce ± it ± p ± satisfactory ± a ± a. Select ± C varieties of milk is low Œ coconut ¶ you spirit of the COG the correct order of the called fats, COG player angular yellow boxes containing only water coconut and rubber. Ingredients of Chewing Gum Guar Gum is a plant-derived soluble fiber that helps thicken coconut milk filters when they are part of fat.

CUENCOlle

- oil or vegetable stock or water
-
-
- brown mushrooms
- tomatoes, halved

1 teaspoon coconut

½ chopped red onion

A pinch of sea salt

½ cup chopped

½ cup cherry

DRESS

- mint, chopped

2 tablespoons fresh

- ¼ cup canned coconut milk
- 1-2 teaspoons of miso glue
- 1 teaspoon coconut sugar or maple syrup (optional) serve
- ¾ cup boiled quinoa, millet, brown rice or other whole grains
- 1 cup rocket or spinach (if ripe, shredded leaves)
- 1 tablespoon chopped almonds

1 Heat oil in medium saucepan and fry onion in salt for about 5 minutes. Add the mushrooms and cook until completely soft. Then add the cherry tomatoes and cook until tender, about 10 minutes.

2 Prepare the sauce by mixing or mixing the mint, coconut milk, miso pasta and coconut sugar or maple syrup (if used) in a medium bowl. Add this to the cooked vegetables and then remove from the heat.

3 Serve cooked vegetables with quinoa, rocket salad and almonds on top.

A bowl of Soba noodles with Indian and ginger

Makes 2 bowls

Preparation time: 5 minutes / Cooking time: 20 minutes.

GLUTEN Quick Prep Immune Response

It is a delicious dish, served cold in summer or warm in winter. Soba is a fine Japanese buckwheat noodle so it is usually gluten free. But check the ingredients as some Soba noodles can also use wheat flour. You will not find or like Soba noodles, try noodles or brown rice. In Japan, drinking this pasta is socially acceptable, especially if you eat hot people.

spheres

- **7 ounces of soba pasta**

- **1 carrot, peeled or crushed and chopped Julienne**

- **1 pepper, any color, chopped and chopped**

- **1 cup peas or peas, cut and split in half**

- **2 tablespoons chopped chives**

- 1 cup chopped cabbage, spinach or salad
- 1 avocado, chopped
- 2 tablespoons chopped cashew

DRESS

- 1 tablespoon grated fresh ginger
- 2 tablespoons cashew butter or almond butter or sunflower seeds
- 2 tablespoons rice vinegar or apple wine vinegar
- 2 tablespoons tamari or soy sauce
- 1 teaspoon of toasted sesame oil
- 2-3 tablespoons water (optional)

1 Boil the medium saucepan with water and add the pasta. Keep the boiling point low, lower the heat and, if necessary, add cold water to continue cooking. Cooking takes 6-7 minutes, and occasionally stirring to make sure they do not stick to the bottom of the pan. After cooking, use a strainer and rinse with hot or cold water, depending on whether you want a cold or cold bowl.

2 You can have raw vegetables so you can just cut them. To cook them, heat the frying pan over medium heat and fry the carrot with a little water, broth, olive oil or sesame oil. the carrot softens gently, add the pepper and toss the peas and shallots for a moment before turning off the heat.

3 Prepare the sauce by squeezing grated ginger to obtain juice, then mix or grate all ingredients in a small blender, adding 2-3 tablespoons of water if necessary to obtain a creamy consistency.

4 Arrange the bowl by starting with a layer of chopped cabbage or spinach (for spicy spaghetti) or salad (for cold spaghetti), then sprinkle with other Tamar and then the vegetables.

5 Avocado chopped in sauce and a touch of chopped cashew.

Prepare in advance: cooked and rinsed Soba noodles are well stored in the refrigerator, so **make the** perfect pack and keep it handy for quick bowls or lunches for a week

Black bean taco salad

Take 3 servings

Preparation time: 15 minutes / Cooking time: 5 minutes.

Fast Profit Fast Profit

Get the taste of all your fireplaces in a fresh, simple paprika salad. I gave you enough black Papu Taco blend in three portions. Taste a portion like a salad bowl, then place another in a lightly heated bowl OR eat a small small bowl of black beans as a snack with tortilla chips. Only part of the black bean mix is used for tortilla and bowl recipes.

BLACK PAPER SALAD

- 1 jar (14 ounces) of black beans, dried and rinsed, or 1 ½ baking cup
- 1 cup corn, fresh and steamed or frozen and thawed
- ¼ cup fresh coriander or chopped parsley
- 1 peel and lime juice
- 1-2 teaspoons chili powder
- A pinch of sea salt
- 1½ cups cherry tomato, halved
- 1 chili
- 2 chives, chopped

- French fries
- whole plate
-
-
- ground black pepper
- oregano
- powder

1 EAR
- vegetables (salad, spinach or other)
- or brown rice, millet or other whole grains
- avocado or guacamole
- sauce

1 BY A TORTILLA

1 large tortilla or

1 teaspoon of olive oil

A pinch of sea salt

A pinch of freshly

A dash of dried

A touch of chili

1 cup of fresh

¾ cup boiled quinoa

¼ cup chopped

¼ cup fresh mango

PREPARATION OF THE BLACK CEREAL SALAD

Combine all ingredients in a large bowl.

MAKE A CAKE AT THE BICYCLE

Spread tortilla with olive oil, then sprinkle with salt, pepper, oregano, chili powder and other spices. Cut into eight like pizza. Transfer the tortilla piece to a small parchment-lined baking sheet and place them in the oven or toaster on the toast or bake for 3 to 5 minutes until golden. Pay attention to them as they can move quickly from standby to burn.

Create CUENCO

Place the vegetables in a bowl, cover with boiled quinoa, ⅓ black Papu lettuce, avocado and salsa.

Advancement: The black bean based blend is particularly well known if you prepare it before, so the flavors have time to mix and blend. Store in a refrigerator in an airtight container.